25

DIAGNOSIS OF
MALARIA

Editors:

Francisco J. López-Antuñano
and
Gabriel Schmunis

PAHO/WHO Communicable Diseases Program

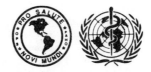

Scientific Publication No. 512

PAN AMERICAN HEALTH ORGANIZATION
Pan American Sanitary Bureau, Regional Office of the
WORLD HEALTH ORGANIZATION
525 Twenty-third Street, N.W.
Washington, DC 20037, USA

1990

Production of this monograph was partially funded by the
United States Agency for International Development

Published also in Spanish (1988) with the title:
Diagnóstico de Malaria
ISBN 92 75 31512 4

First Reprint, 1994

ISBN 92 75 11512 5

AUTHORS

DR. RICHARD L. BEAUDOIN, Malaria Division, Naval Medical Research Institute, Bethesda, MD, United States of America

DR. MARCOS BOULOS, Malaria Laboratory, Superintendency of Control of Endemias, São Paulo, SP, Brazil

DR. ANTONIO WALTER FERREIRA, Seroepidemiology Laboratory, Institute of Tropical Medicine, Faculty of Medicine, University of São Paulo, São Paulo, SP, Brazil

DR. ROBERT W. GWADZ, Medical Entomology Unit, Malaria Section, Laboratory of Parasitic Diseases, National Institute of Allergy and Infectious Diseases, National Institutes of Health, Bethesda, MD, United States of America

DR. FRANCISCO J. LÓPEZ-ANTUÑANO, Communicable Diseases Program, Pan American Health Organization, Washington, DC, United States of America

DR. JANINE M. RAMSEY, Communicable Diseases Program, Pan American Health Organization, Tapachula, Chiapas, Mexico

DR. VIRGILIO DO ROSARIO, Biomedical Research Institute, Rockville, MD, United States of America

DR. FIDEL ZAVALA, Department of Medical and Molecular Parasitology, New York University Medical Center, New York, NY, United States of America

CONTENTS

PREFACE

Vector-borne diseases, such as malaria, represent a menace to the health of a large portion of the population in developing countries. In order to gain an understanding of the epidemiology of malaria as a social and biomedical problem and of its impact on the development of health systems, it is imperative that the infection be diagnosed accurately and promptly.

One of the Pan American Health Organization's strategic priorities is the dissemination of scientific and technical information, especially as it relates to advances achieved through health research. The *Manual for the Microscopic Diagnosis of Malaria* was first published in 1960, and it was so well received that three additional, updated editions had been produced by 1973. Recently, there has been great demand for a manual that would bring together the most current knowledge about the biology of plasmodia, their behavior in their anopheline vectors, and human response to infection. The present monograph has been prepared to answer that need, and it constitutes an expanded and up-to-date diagnostic tool.

The attempt has been made to assure that the principles and recommendations relating to the diagnostic methods are described clearly and simply. The goal is not only the uniform application of these diagnostic techniques by specialized malaria prevention and control programs but also their efficient incorporation into general health services.

As local health systems are strengthened and become better developed and organized, more and better diagnostic services will be required. We hope this publication will make a substantial contribution towards their operation.

CARLYLE GUERRA DE MACEDO
DIRECTOR

Chapter 1

LIFE CYCLE I.
THE EXOERYTHROCYTIC STAGES OF MALARIA PARASITES IN HUMANS

Richard L. Beaudoin

Although the parasites infecting human red blood cells were discovered over a century ago by Laveran (1), awareness of the existence of the preerythrocytic stage in the liver did not occur until relatively recently (2). Today, the tissue stage remains the least understood of any part of the plasmodial life cycle in man. However, during the last 10 years there has been a renewed interest in exoerythrocytic parasites, and they are now center stage in one of the most exciting and imaginative dramas being played out in the continuing story of malaria research.

Despite their importance in establishing the first foothold of infection in man and the role they play in providing a source of renewed parasitemias or relapses, parasites in the exoerythrocytic or liver stage are not readily detected by routine microscopic or serologic procedures. Consequently, they are not presently considered to have diagnostic value.

BIOLOGY

The term exoerythrocytic refers to the stage of the parasite that does not take place in human erythrocytes. This stage is nonpigmented, since the plasmodia infect liver parenchymal cells, where they do not use hemoglobin. This distinguishes it from the erythrocytic stage, in which the plasmodia, including gametocytes, infect circulating erythrocytes where they produce malarial pigment, or hemozoin. The precise way in which sporozoites inoculated into man by the mosquito reach hepatocytes and become established in them is not yet well understood.

The classical theory of exoerythrocytic development was that of a cyclical schizogony in the liver parenchymal cells similar to the schizogonic development that occurs in red blood cells. According to this concept, the sporozoite is inoculated into the capillary system by a mosquito during a blood meal. It is then carried to the liver by the bloodstream and manages to establish itself in a hepatocyte, where it begins to develop and multiply asexually. Eventually, mature schizonts are formed and exoerythrocytic merozoites are released. The latter then invade either a red blood cell, thereby initiating the erythrocytic cycle, or another hepatocyte, continuing the liver cycle.

This classical theory of a continuing cycle in the liver was especially attractive, since it offered an explanation of the phenomenon of relapse, a characteristic of some forms of the disease. Moreover, the cyclical development concept was strongly supported by direct evidence from avian malaria, where proof of continuous exoerythrocytic schizogony was already available. However, the general hypothesis had to be modified to accommodate the peculiarities of the four species of *Plasmodium* infecting man. For instance, it has long been known that *P. falciparum* infections do not relapse, since a radical cure is achieved when the erythrocytic parasites are eliminated following treatment with chloroquine or quinine, although neither of these antimalarials is known to exert any effect on the liver stage (3).

It had also been shown that *P. malariae* infections in human volunteers could be radically cured by chloroquine, which suggested these infections likewise lacked a continuous liver cycle. These observations and others (4) have led in recent years to a revision of the cyclical theory of exoerythrocytic development. Presently, continuous exoerythrocytic development is believed to be restricted to *P. vivax* and *P. ovale*; however, alternative explanations of secondary development in the liver are still being sought for these two species. One of the alternatives that has received attention proposes that latent stages exist which are responsible for relapses (5). This idea has culminated in formulation of the hypnozoite theory, which postulates the existence of discrete subpopulations of sporozoites that give rise to equally discrete subpopulations of exoerythrocytic trophozoites. Thus, a single inoculation by a mosquito of sporozoites of a relapsing malaria theoretically contains a mixture of genetically distinct parasites in sufficient numbers to provide for the relapse pattern characteristic of the strain. Some of these trophozoite subpopulations develop immediately, while others lie dormant for varying periods of time. These dormant trophozoite forms have been named hypnozoites; according to the theory, it is their "awakening" and subsequent development to maturity, ending with release of merozoites into the circulation, that accounts for relapses (6).

This hypothesis holds that all sporozoites reach the target host cell, enter it, and transform into uninucleate trophozoites at the same time. Some develop immediately into mature schizonts. Others, the hypnozoites, remain dormant for prespecified periods of time ranging from weeks to months. The period of dormancy varies with the subpopulation and is believed to be a genetically determined intrinsic property of the parasite (6, 7). Although the hypnozoite theory is gaining acceptance, the existence of hypnozoites and their biological significance to malaria relapse are subjects that are still debated by some malariologists (8–10), as will be discussed in more detail later in this chapter.

In summary, the exoerythrocytic cycle of the nonrelapsing species of *Plasmodium* infecting humans is believed to consist of a single preerythrocytic cycle in the liver culminating in the release of a large number of merozoites that invade only red blood cells. Following the rupture of these preerythrocytic schizonts, no further parasites remain in the liver cells. *P. falciparum* and *P. malariae* follow this pattern. In contrast, relapsing species have persistent liver stages, which are the source of the parasites that cause relapses. These forms are thought by some to be produced continuously by secondary cycling in hepatocytes, whereas others believe that hypnozoites are responsible for relapses. *P. vivax* and *P. ovale* are the two species infecting man that produce relapses.

NONRELAPSING MALARIAS

PLASMODIUM FALCIPARUM

There is general agreement that a single preerythrocytic stage occurs in this species. The primary attack follows initial exoerythrocytic development, after which no exoerythrocytic parasites remain in the liver. True relapses do not occur in infections with this species, and recurrences of detectable blood forms after periods of apparent latency are referred to as recrudescences, although the terminology is disputed by some (11).

Probably the most accurate estimate of the length of development of the primary liver stage in humans of *P. falciparum* was obtained by Fairley for New Guinea isolates of that species (12). Volunteers from the Australian army were inoculated with sporozoites by mosquito bite, and then the infected volunteers were monitored for circulating parasites in their blood. The parasites were detected by subinoculation of 500 ml of the volunteers' blood at regular intervals into a second group of volunteers who had never had malaria, to test the blood's infectiousness. The subinoculations were infective to the second group of volunteers when done with blood taken less than one hour after the bites on the first volunteers, that is, while the sporozoites were still circulating in the peripheral blood. No infective forms of the parasite were found circulating in the donors between one hour and five days after the bites of infected mosquitoes, indicating that complete development in the liver requires about five days for this strain.

Another study, based on observations of 220 patients, reported an average prepatent period of 11 days following naturally induced infections with six different strains (13). Complete development—from inoculation of sporozoites to release of exoerythrocytic merozoites—would have required about nine days, assuming that a minimum of two days was needed to produce a detectable parasitemia once merozoites were released into the bloodstream. However, in this same study a prepatent period as short as six days was recorded for two patients, and one patient had a prepatent period that extended to 25 days. This indicates that under certain conditions considerable variation may exist in the time required for exoerythrocytic development, although in the case of the last patient, the possibility of resistance of the red blood cells to infection cannot be entirely dismissed.

The time frame of six days agrees well with the direct observations of Shortt *et al.* (14). Mosquitoes infected with a Romanian strain fed on a human volunteer who five-and-a-half days later had a piece of liver removed by laparotomy. Histopathologic examination of the liver fragment revealed mature exoerythrocytic schizonts in the parenchymal cells; subinoculation of the first patient's blood to a second volunteer at this time produced infection in the recipient. Shortly thereafter, this experiment was replicated by Jeffery *et al.* using a Central American strain of the parasite (15), for which a prepatent period of seven days was found.

The exoerythrocytic development of a Liberian strain of *P. falciparum* inoculated into chimpanzees was studied by Bray (16). His report gives a detailed description of the entire cycle, beginning with the early binucleate parasite measuring 4 μm in diameter two days after inoculation, and continuing through completion of schizogony when thousands of merozoites are visible. In the chimpanzee, the process requires a slightly longer time than it does in man. Exoerythrocytic schizogony of *P. falciparum* differs from schizogony in the liver stage of the other human plasmodia by the occurrence in this species of a process called aposchizogony *(16)*. In aposchizogony, the schizont grows until it reaches a diameter of about 30 μm, which in man occurs by day four and in the chimpanzee on day five. At this point, the parasite is still rounded-to-oval, with a smooth, regular contour. By the following day, however, the schizont has divided into numerous cytomeres, which consist of a large central vacuole surrounded by a periplast lined with nuclei. These cytomeres are the result of rapid division of a large, multinucleate syncytium likewise containing a central vacuole. As division proceeds, each cytomere becomes smaller and contains progressively fewer nuclei, until uninucleate merozoites are formed.

In man, the mature exoerythrocytic schizont of *P. falciparum* measures about 60 μm and produces an estimated 30,000 merozoites *(17)*.

PLASMODIUM MALARIAE

The exoerythrocytic development of *P. malariae* is not as well studied as that of either *P. falciparum* or *P. vivax*, in part because of difficulty in obtaining mosquitoes infected with only *P. malariae* *(13, 17)*, since this species is most frequently encountered in nature in a mixed infection, and also because of difficulty in infecting many strains of laboratory mosquitoes with it. Thus, any conclusions are drawn from very few data gleaned from a restricted number of naturally transmitted human cases. Nonetheless, the available data indicate that the length of time required to complete schizogonic development in the liver is appreciably longer for *P. malariae* than for the other species of human plasmodia.

The period required to complete liver schizogony in man varies from 21 to 31 days. This estimate is based on a prepatent period ranging from 27 to 37 days and assumes two subpatent blood cycles of three days each prior to patency *(13)*.

Bray *(18)*, on the other hand, found *P. malariae* in chimpanzee erythrocytes only 16 days after mosquito inoculation of sporozoites, while Ciuca *et al.* *(19)* reported detecting blood stages in man as early as 18 days following sporozoite inoculation of the VS strain of *P. malariae*. Graham *(17)*, also working with this strain, induced an infection in a neurosyphilitic patient by sporozoite inoculation and subsequently used blood from this patient to inoculate five other neurosyphilitic patients on days 13, 14, 15, 16, and 17. Transmission of the infection to the recipients was the criterion for proving circulating blood parasites in the donor. The recipients subinoculated on days 15 and 17 both became patent, demonstrating that the period required to complete exoerythrocytic development, at least for the VS strain, was no greater than 15 days.

It is possible that the discrepancy between prepatent periods observed in man by different authors reflects a wide variation in exoerythrocytic development time between strains of this species. The small number of cases studied does not shed much light on this point and, unfortunately, direct observations of exoerythrocytic development of *P. malariae* in humans are not available.

Liver stages of *P. malariae* were observed directly in liver sections from chimpanzees *(18)*, in which the nearly mature liver schizont contained about 1,500 nuclei at 12 days. Garnham estimated that approximately 2,000 merozoites are produced by each exoerythrocytic schizont of *P. malariae* *(17)*. He observed an aggregation of vacuoles around the periphery of the schizont. These vacuoles grow with the parasite to a diameter of 5 to 8 μm each, at which point they appear orange in color. At 12 days, when the schizont measures about 41 μm, it begins to develop pronounced lobulation and vacuolation, suggesting that the exoerythrocytic schizont does not mature in the chimpanzee until after 13 days (17).

Because sporozoite-induced infections of P. malariae can be cured with blood schizonticidal drugs, it is believed that neither hypnozoite nor secondary exoerythrocytic forms of this species of malaria parasite persist.

RELAPSING MALARIAS

PLASMODIUM VIVAX

The preerythrocytic liver stages of P. vivax, like those of P. falciparum, have been relatively well studied, and the details of primary development are known. Based on results from a study of 428 natural infections with nine different strains of P. vivax, prepatent periods range from 8 to 23 days, with a mean of 12.2 (20). A period of from 6 to 21 days with a mean 10.2 days would be required to complete exoerythrocytic schizogony in the liver cell, assuming, as with P. falciparum, the need for a minimum of one complete, 48-hour erythrocytic cycle following release of the exoerythrocytic merozoites to achieve a parasite density sufficient to be detectable in stained thick blood films.

The minimum time required for exoerythrocytic development in man of P. vivax was most precisely established in experiments that used an approach identical to the one used for P. falciparum (12). Blood from infected patients was systematically subinoculated into uninfected volunteers at intervals of minutes to days after the donor had received the infective sporozoite inoculum from a mosquito. Recipients of the subinoculated blood were then monitored to establish the period of time between disappearance of sporozoites from the circulation and the appearance of the erythrocytic stage. The results suggested that the period required for P. vivax to complete exoerythrocytic development is about eight days.

This estimate of the time required to complete the primary cycle agrees closely with direct observations made on human liver biopsies taken by laparotomy (21) (Figure 1.1), in which mature schizonts were found eight days after inoculation with infective sporozoites. Bray (22) reported similar results for sporozoite-induced infections in chimpanzees. Based on these microscopic observations, it has been estimated that approximately 10,000 merozoites are produced by a single preerythrocytic schizont.

As already discussed, experimental studies on human volunteers have indicated that blood schizonticides do not sterilize an infection produced by either P. vivax or P. ovale, since parasitemia will reappear following elimination of the primary erythrocytic infection by chloroquine or quinine. This is in contrast to blood-induced infections with P. falciparum and P. malariae, which are radically cured with either of these antimalarials. By convention, malariologists working on human plasmodia have restricted the term relapse to recurrences originating from parasites in host liver cells. As pointed out in the section on nonrelapsing malaria, recurrences in P. falciparum and P. malariae originate from subpatent blood infections and are referred

to as recrudescences. Although there is still dispute over the preferred terminology
(11), the main issue to be resolved is the nature of the forms in the liver that give
rise to renewed blood infections known as relapses following chloroquine treatment.
Two alternative explanations for the origin of these recurrences have been proposed:
the classical cycling theory and the hypnozoite theory.

The classical cycling theory holds that preerythrocytic schizogony is followed
by reinvasion of liver cells by some first generation exoerythrocytic merozoites, while
other progeny of this same brood invade red blood cells. Relapses are the product
of renewed erythrocyte invasion by merozoites produced by secondary schizogony
that follows periods of latency after the primary attack has subsided and during which
existing immunity has waned. This theory does not provide any compelling reasons
for the occurrence of different periods of time between relapses in infection with
different strains, nor does it provide a satisfactory explanation for long prepatent
periods. Furthermore, the many relapse patterns observed in different strains are
not adequately explained on the basis of variable immune states.

The hypnozoite theory, on the other hand, suggests that recurrences of parasitemia are actually brought about by spontaneous development of schizonts from
latent uninucleate forms in the liver called hypnozoites. These forms are thought to
be genetically programmed to continue their development at a predetermined time,
completing schizogony and releasing waves of merozoites into the bloodstream. These
merozoites then go on to invade reticulocytes, thereby initiating the first relapse or
what amounts to a delayed, second erythrocytic attack. The next recurrence would
then really be a third attack after a longer delay, and so on. Thus, it would be possible
to experience a large number of successive erythrocytic attacks originating from the
original inoculum of sporozoites and not from a secondary schizogonic cycle in the
liver in infections with either *P. vivax* or *P. ovale*. These recurrences would result
from a series of schizogonies, each of which would produce a progressively delayed
attack. As stated previously, the hypothesis maintains that the period of latency is
under genetic control (7) and that each inoculum of *P. vivax* sporozoites consists of
a mixture of genetically distinct sporozoite subpopulations, distinguished from the
others by the length of delay of trophozoite (=hypnozoite) development.

Evidence cited in favor of the hypothesis is the existence of strain differences
with respect to prepatent period and relapse pattern. For purposes of comparison,
two very different patterns will be discussed. The first pattern is exemplified by the
Chesson strain from New Guinea, which has a short incubation period of about 13
days and therefore probably requires only seven to eight days to complete primary
schizogonic development in the liver. Following the primary attack, parasitemias
recur at intervals of two to three months for a period of up to two years (23).

The other pattern is displayed by strains with "long" incubation periods and
variable recurrence patterns. The incubation periods vary from long (*hiberans* strain
from northern Russia, after which the group is named), frequently prolonged (Ca-
meroons strain), occasionally long (MS (Moscow) and Dutch), to much shorter (Mad-
agascar and St. Elizabeth strains), and the latent periods between recurrences are
long (17). On the basis of these characteristics and others, the two groups were
judged sufficiently different to justify their separation into two subspecies, *P. vivax
vivax* and *P. vivax hibernans* (24). Recently, a third subspecies has been added,
P. vivax multinucleatum (25).

In the Americas, the interval between the primary attack and the first relapse varies from five to ten months, based on observations of patients infected with strains from El Salvador, Nicaragua, Panama, and Venezuela (26).

To be consistent with the hypnozoite hypothesis, the group of parasites collectively classified as *P. vivax* would have to be considered a complex consisting of a large number of genetically distinct parasite subpopulations. This in turn would require that the genes controlling the incubation period and duration of latency be included in each inoculum of sporozoites that the vector receives in a blood meal. Otherwise, strains would not consistently exhibit their characteristic relapse patterns in the vertebrate host. The hypothesis must also adequately explain how a mosquito, which usually lives only a few weeks, can consistently pick up a sufficiently diverse panel of gametocytes to provide the gene pool responsible for recurrences that can happen in the human host over a two-year period. Furthermore, the mosquito would have to consistently transmit this complete assortment of genes—each variety packaged in its own sporozoite—with the single inoculum it delivers to the vertebrate host when it transmits the infection. This would appear to be a formidable assignment, requiring that the mosquito infected by feeding on gametocytes derived from one particular hypnozoite "subpopulation" (e.g., the "third relapse subpopulation") be able to pick up in a single blood meal at least one gametocyte pair carrying the genes coding for the primary and each of the subsequent relapse subpopulations characteristic of the strain. Every mosquito transmitting the infection, therefore, would consistently have to have had a minimum number of oocysts corresponding to at least one half of the "relapse" subpopulations, since each oocyst, although derived from a single diploid zygote, is haploid. Admittedly, the hypnozoite hypothesis is both imaginative and exciting, and it may well be correct. However, it must address questions relating to the issues raised here and elsewhere (27) before accounts of the life cycle of the relapsing malaria parasites are rewritten to reflect it.

PLASMODIUM OVALE

James *et al.* (27) reported the mean incubation period for mosquito-induced infections of *Plasmodium ovale* in 36 nonimmune volunteers as 13.6 days. Assuming one erythrocytic cycle of two days to reach patency and an additional two-day cycle to obtain a density sufficient to bring about onset of clinical symptoms, the length of time required to complete liver schizogony would be 9.6 days. However, delayed primary attacks of up to 19 months have been encountered with this parasite.

The blood stages of *Plasmodium ovale* are so similar to those of *P. vivax* that, in light infections, it is often difficult even for experienced malaria microscopists to differentiate the two with certainty. In geographic areas where both species exist, conservative malariologists will often classify an infection as *vivax/ovale* rather than risk a mistaken diagnosis. However, unlike the blood stage, the liver stage of *P. ovale* is readily distinguishable by parasite morphology and by the extent of the distortion caused to the infected parenchymal cell (29).

When development of the liver stage of *P. ovale* was studied in sections of liver fragments surgically removed from an infected volunteer, it was found that schizogony was completed in about nine days. The morphology of this parasite is strikingly different from all other exoerythrocytic forms of plasmodia in the size of the trophozoite nucleus, in the distortion the parasite causes to the parenchymal cell (especially the hypertrophy of its nucleus), and finally in the huge size of the lobulated schizont stage, which can measure 70–80 μm by 50 μm with a volume estimated at 123,940 μm^3. The number of merozoites in a schizont of this size was reported to be 15,443, and the merozoites were also uncommonly large, each measuring about 1.8 μm in diameter (29).

Blood infection recurrences originating from liver forms are common with this parasite and can correctly be termed relapses, keeping in mind the same caveats that were discussed in the section on *P. vivax*.

REFERENCES

(1) Laveran, A. Note sure un nouveau parasite trouvé dans le sang de plusieurs malades atteints de fievre palustre. *Bull Acad Natl Med (Paris)* 9:1235–1236, 1880.

(2) Shortt, H. E., and P. C. C. Garnham. Pre-erythrocytic stage in mammalian malaria parasites. *Nature* 161:126, 1948.

(3) Covell, G., G. R. Coatney, J. W. Field, and J. Singh. *Chemotherapy of Malaria*. Monogr. Ser. 27. Geneva: World Health Organization, 1955.

(4) Coatney, G. R., W. E. Collins, McW. Warren, and P. G. Contacos. *The Primate Malarias*. Washington: U.S. Government Printing Office, 1971.

(5) Shute, P. G. Latency and long-term relapse in benign tertian malaria. *Trans R Soc Trop Med Hyg* 40:189–200, 1946.

(6) Krotoski, W. A. Discovery of the hypnozoite and a new theory of malarial relapse. *Trans R Soc Trop Med Hyg* 79:1–11, 1985.

(7) Krotoski, W. A., R. S. Bray, P. C. C. Garnham, R. W. Gwadz, R. Killick-Kendrick, C. C. Draper, G. A. T. Targett, D. M. Krotoski, M. W. Guy, L. C. Koontz, and F. B. Cogswell. Observations on early and late post-sporozoite tissue stages in primate malaria. II. The hypnozoite of *Plasmodium cynomolgi bastianellii* from 3 to 105 days after infection, and detection of 36- to 40-hour preerythrocytic forms. *Am J Trop Med Hyg* 31:211–225, 1982.

(8) Shortt, H. E. Relapse in primate malaria: Its implications for the disease in man. *Trans R Soc Trop Med Hyg* 77:734–736, 1983.

(9) Corradetti, A. About the hypnozoites of the *vivax*-like group of *Plasmodia*. *Trans R Soc Trop Med Hyg* 79:879–880, 1985.

(10) Krotoski, W. A. About the hypnozoites of the *vivax*-like group of *Plasmodia*: A reply. *Trans R Soc Trop Med Hyg* 79:880, 1985.

(11) Bruce-Chwatt, L. J. Terminology of relapsing malaria: Enigma variations. *Trans R Soc Trop Med Hyg* 78:844–845, 1984.

(12) Fairley, N. H. Sidelights on malaria in man obtained by subinoculation experiments. *Trans R Soc Trop Med Hyg* 40:621–676, 1947.

(13) Kitchen, S. F. Symptomatology: General Considerations. Chapter 40 *in*: M. F. Boyd (ed.), *Malariology*, Vol. II: Intermediate Host. Philadelphia and London: W. B. Saunders Company, 1949.

(14) Shortt, H. E., N. H. Fairley, G. Covell, P. G. Shute, and P. C. C. Garnham. The pre-erythrocytic stage of *Plasmodium falciparum*. *Trans R Soc Trop Med Hyg* 44:405–419, 1951.

(15) Jeffery, G. M., G. B. Wolcott, M. D. Young, and D. Williams. Exoerythrocytic stages of *Plasmodium falciparum*. *Am J Trop Med Hyg* 1:917–926, 1952.

(16) Bray, R. S. Observations on the cytology and morphology of the mammalian malaria parasites. I. A process of apparent plasmotomy in the pre-erythrocytic phase of *Laverania falcipara*. *Rev Parasitol* 21:267–276, 1960.

(17) Garnham, P. C. C. *Malaria Parasites and Other Haemosporidia*. Oxford: Blackwell Scientific Publications, 1966.

(18) Bray, R. S. Studies on malaria in chimpanzees. VIII. The experimental transmission and pre-erythrocytic phase of *Plasmodium malariae* with a note on the host range of the parasite. *Am J Trop Med Hyg* 9:455–465, 1960.

(19) Ciuca, M., G. Lupascu, E. Negulici, and P. Constantinescu. Recherches sur la transmission experimental de *P. malariae* à l'homme. *Arch Roum Path Exp Microbiol* 23:763–776, 1964.

(20) Kitchen, S. F. *Vivax* malaria. Chapter 43 *in*: M. F. Boyd (ed.), *Malariology*, Vol. II: Intermediate Host. Philadelphia and London: W. B. Saunders Company, 1949.

(21) Shortt, H. E., and P. C. C. Garnham. The pre-erythrocytic development of *Plasmodium cynomolgi* and *Plasmodium vivax*. *Trans R Soc Trop Med Hyg* 41:785–795, 1948.

(22) Bray, R. S. Studies on malaria in chimpanzees. II. *Plasmodium vivax. Am J Trop Med Hyg* 6:514–519, 1957.

(23) Coatney, G. R., W. C. Cooper, and M. D. Young. Studies in human malaria. XXX. A summary of 204 sporozoite-induced infections with the Chesson strain of *Plasmodium vivax. J Natl Malar Soc* 9:381–396, 1950.

(24) Nikolaiev, B. P. Subspecies of the parasite of tertian malaria (*Plasmodium vivax*). *Dokl Akad Nauk SSSR* 67:201–210. Cited from P. C. C. Garnham, *Malaria Parasites and Other Haemosporidia.* Oxford: Blackwell Scientific Publications, 1966.

(25) Jiang, J. B., J. C. Huang, D. S. Liang, J. X. Liu, S. W. Zhang, and F. C. Cheng. Long incubation of *Plasmodium vivax multinucleatum* as demonstrated in 3 experimental human cases. *Trans R Soc Trop Med Hyg* 76:845–847, 1982.

(26) Contacos, P. G., W. E. Collins, G. M. Jeffery, W. A. Krotoski, and W. A. Howard. Studies on the characterization of *Plasmodium vivax* strains from Central America. *Am J Trop Med Hyg* 21:707–712, 1972.

(27) Schmidt, L. H. Compatibility of relapse patterns of *Plasmodium cynomolgi* infections in rhesus monkeys with continuous cyclical development and hypnozoite concepts of relapse. *Am J Trop Med Hyg* 35:1077–1099, 1986.

(28) James, S. P., W. D. Nicol, and P. G. Shute. *Ovale* malaria. Chapter 44 *in*: M. F. Boyd (ed.), *Malariology*, Vol. II: Intermediate Host. Philadelphia and London: W. B. Saunders Company, 1949.

(29) Garnham, P. C. C., R. S. Bray, W. Cooper, R. Lainson, F. I. Awad, and J. Williamson. The pre-erythrocytic stage of *Plasmodium ovale. Trans R Soc Trop Med Hyg* 49:158–167, 1955.

Chapter 2

LIFE CYCLE II. THE ERYTHROCYTIC CYCLE OF MALARIA IN HUMANS

Virgilio do Rosario

Patients usually first seek treatment for malaria owing to clinical symptoms that appear when the parasites invade their erythrocytes. Diagnosis is carried out in the laboratory by microscopic visualization of parasites in stained blood smears (1, 2). Descriptions of the morphologies of the four human malaria parasites (*Plasmodium falciparum*, *P. vivax*, *P. malariae*, and *P. ovale*) and of the symptoms observed in patients carrying these parasites are contained in other chapters of this monograph. A trained person can distinguish the different types of human malaria parasites based only on the morphology of the ring stage (Figures 2.1 and 2.2), although this is not necessarily easy and may give rise to diagnostic errors (3). Other diagnosis techniques, such as DNA probes, may help overcome this problem (4, 5).

Asexual reproduction of malarial parasites in the human host begins in the parenchymal cells of the liver (exoerythrocytic cycle) and continues in the red blood cells (erythrocytic cycle). *P. falciparum* causes malignant tertian malaria, "tertian" meaning that every third day the merozoites invade the red blood cells and reinitiate an erythrocytic cycle (merozoite-ring stage-trophozoite-schizont-merozoite). Other malarial parasites that also have a 48-hour development period are *P. vivax* (which causes benign tertian malaria) and *P. ovale* (which causes ovale tertian malaria). The other human malaria parasite, *P. malariae*, has a longer cycle that lasts 72 hours. It is responsible for benign quartan malaria—that is, the patient presents symptoms every fourth day. Figures 2.1 to 2.4 illustrate these different parasites at different stages.

Theoretically, parasites of any of these four species can develop simultaneously in the same patient. In practice, infections by more than two species at a time are not observed; the infecting species can be differentiated by careful microscopic examination of blood smears. Clinical observations over the years have shown that the different species of malaria parasites cause different symptoms. Also, it is well known that *P. falciparum* has only one cycle in the liver prior to the erythrocytic cycle. For *P. vivax* and *P. ovale*, there is evidence that some parasites remain in the liver as latent forms (hypnozoites), while for *P. malariae*, a reduced number of parasites can remain over a long time period in the red blood cells. This chapter, however, will concentrate on the differences that exist between parasites belonging to the same species.

It took many more years to detect chloroquine resistance in *P. falciparum* in Africa than in Asia or South America (6–8), which implied the existence of variation between the parasites from these different geographic regions. Within a given region, it frequently happens that a person presents with more than one attack of *falciparum* malaria within a limited time period. Two reasons can be proposed to explain this:

a) the patient was exposed to a new inoculation of sporozoites, by mosquito bite, giving rise to a new successive infection, or b) the new malaria infection is caused by a population of blood-stage parasites that resisted the patient's immune response or the drug treatment that was administered to the patient (a recrudescent infection). One malaria infection does not automatically induce in the human host an immune response that will protect the patient against infection by other, genetically different parasites of the same *Plasmodium* species. In the case of *P. vivax*, the repeated parasitemias in the same host may also be due to dormant liver-stage forms that eventually produce merozoites (relapse infection).

Routine tests, such as microscopic observation of stained, uncloned parasites, although clinically important, give little information on the diversity of parasite populations in a patient (9). Since laboratory-based biological and biochemical characterization studies usually require large quantities of parasites, few such studies could be done before the advent of *in vitro* culture of *P. falciparum* (10). With that technique, large amounts of parasite material can be produced quickly, enabling such studies. Table 2.1 gives some guidelines for identifying parasites in mixed infections, as well as criteria for identification of possible changes in clones started from isolates.

This chapter will describe how studies carried out with the parasites in the erythrocytic cycle have changed some previously held ideas about malaria. The new concepts these studies have provided for identifying parasites can be of help in the control of the disease.

It is necessary to define some of the terms that will be used. *Diversity* (or variety) among parasites within the same species means parasites that differ in some of their biological and/or biochemical characteristics (for example, drug susceptibility or enzyme types). Often, the term *variation* has been used to express the same meaning, but it also refers to the changes (usually unstable) that homogeneous parasite populations (derived from a clone) exhibit in response to some stimulus or pressure. For example, antigenic variation is a process by which an infectious organism periodically changes the constituent antigenic molecules exposed on its surface in order to avoid elimination by the host's immune system (11). This has been observed in African trypanosomes and has only recently been confirmed for *P. falciparum* (11, 12).

The term *isolate* refers to the parasites collected from a single patient at one given time. If blood is taken from the same patient again, even on the same day,

Table 2.1. Criteria for the identification of parasites in mixed infections and in clones obtained from isolates.

In isolates/strains:

a) Different species of malaria parasites, for example, *P. falciparum* and *P. vivax* (visible by microscopy)
b) Same species, different stages of growth (visible by microscopy)
c) Same species, same stage of growth (e.g., rings) distinguished only by specific characterization techniques

In clones (produced in vitro from isolates):

a) Changes in cloned lines may be due to host immune selective pressure (antigenic variation)
b) Changes may be induced by external factors *in vitro*, e.g., mutagenic factors
In both cases a) and b), the parasites can only be distinguished by specific characterization techniques.

the parasites collected will have to be identified as a different sample, due to potential fluctuations in their population. The parasites a patient carries may originate from one single mosquito bite, but that bite can inject a large number of sporozoites. Since genetic recombination occurs prior to the development of sporozoites within the oocyst, one can assume that variation exists among sporozoites from a single mosquito, even if only one female gametocyte was fertilized by one male gametocyte. Therefore, there is the potential for a very diverse, heterogeneous parasite population to exist in the same host, given, for example, the probability of more than one oocyst per mosquito and more than one infective bite per host. The word *strain* is often used as equivalent to isolate. *Line* usually refers to an isolate/strain maintained in continuous *in vitro* culture in the laboratory, or, in the case of rodent malaria parasites, maintained by continuous blood passaging in mice. A *clone* represents a homogeneous parasite population produced from a single parasite. It is obtained by isolating individual parasites by a dilution technique *(13)* or by micromanipulation *(14)* and allowing them to grow. At least two weeks are usually required for development in blood culture. Since homogeneous populations of parasites (clones) do not represent the *in vivo* situation, the practicality of producing these parasites for research is open to question. This subject will be discussed later.

BIOLOGICAL CHARACTERIZATION

No major morphological differences distinguish parasites within the same species. When *P. falciparum* parasites are isolated from a patient to establish an *in vitro* culture, not all of the ring stage forms collected mature into schizonts at the same time. Careful observation of the original stained smear of the patient's blood often shows that the ring forms vary in size, which represents a difference in their stage of development, better studied *in vitro*. It is possible to synchronize parasites' development in culture and compare, for example, the growth cycles of clones obtained from the same isolate. A difference of up to eight hours in the completion of a cycle (ring form to ring form) has been seen. It is interesting to speculate on how these differences in cycle length may affect a factor such as drug action on the parasite. It can also be observed *in vitro* that the number of merozoites within a schizont varies, which means that not all parasites multiply at the same rate; for example, one schizont may produce only 16 nucleii (representing 16 new merozoites and future rings) compared to another that produces 24.

In vitro growth rate studies are not easy to carry out and attempts to correlate such data with the *in vivo* situation are subject to criticism, since results may be affected by the type and age of red blood cells used in culture. In addition, there is an absence of either cellular or humoral immunity against these blood-stage forms in *in vitro* culture work, since only fresh, nonimmune serum is used as an additive to the culture medium. But many factors other than immunity may also affect growth of parasites *in vivo*. Predilection for young red blood cells has been reported for *P. ovale* and *P. vivax*, in contrast to the case for *P. malariae*. It has been suggested that the "Duffy" factor could explain the absence of *P. vivax* in West Africa, where most of the human population is "Duffy"-negative *(15)*. Other evidence indicates that invasion of erythrocytes by merozoites of *P. vivax* appears to occur at sites other than those of the Duffy blood group antigens Fy^a and Fy^b *(16)*. Type of hemoglobin affects infection with *P. falciparum*. Also, the presence or absence of the enzyme G-6-PD and other red blood cell enzymes alters the growth of parasites, and the presence of receptors on the surface of red blood cells alters the merozoite's ability to invade the cells. Data on receptors are far from definitive (17–19). Retardation of development of *P. falciparum* parasites (detected in culture) may also be related to non-antibody factors in the serum, such as one called the "crisis-form factor" (20). This factor was found in serum of Sudanese origin, but not in material obtained from Indonesia. However, although these variables may explain the absence of malaria parasites or inhibition of their invasion and growth in specific individuals, most human beings are still susceptible to the disease.

A recent study (21) showed that absence of a particular gene (marked by a histidine-rich protein, HRP-3) was associated with low growth rate. Although virulence of these parasites is an important characteristic, gametocyte production and the capability of transmission are also areas of concern.

Gametocyte production is now feasible in the laboratory (22). It has been shown that, under standardized conditions, clones from the same isolate show differing abilities to infect mosquitoes (23). Important studies on the capacity of parasites to infect different vector species can now be carried out (24); it has already been shown that some parasite species are only transmitted by one vector even when other potential vectors are present in the area (25).

A number of different models exist for the production of gametocytes. Several factors that induce or affect their production have been described, for example, the immune status of the host and the presence or absence of pressure induced either by drugs, poor nutrient levels, or the presence of parasite-derived metabolites (26, 27). In *P. falciparum* infections, gametocytogenesis has been observed to occur over very prolonged periods of time, either because the patients were infected with genetically different parasites or because they were infected sequentially by repeated mosquito bites. It has been shown (28) that the same schizont was capable of producing both asexual and sexual forms, and that clones from the same isolate do not all have the same infective capability, at least *in vitro* (23). The example in Table 2.2 shows the possibilities of different characteristics that exist among clones from the same isolate. It suggests the situation that may occur in the field in patients with infections by different parasite genotypes within the same parasite species.

Table 2.2. Selection of different populations of *P. falciparum* according to different selective pressures, and their effect on transmission of the infection.[a]

			Transmission in:	
Clone type	Response to chloroquine	Production of gametocytes	Presence of chloroquine	Absence of chloroquine
A	Resistant	NO	NO	NO
B	Sensitive	YES	NO	YES
C	Resistant	YES	YES	YES

[a] If a patient has these three different parasite populations, subpopulation A will never be transmitted, since it does not produce gametocytes. Although it infected this patient, for unknown reasons the subpopulation has lost the capability of transmission. Subpopulations B and C will survive if no treatment is given. However, with treatment, only subpopulation C will survive and thus only that parasite population can transmit the infection.

BIOCHEMICAL CHARACTERIZATION

Enzyme typing of malaria parasites has been done on rodent malaria models (29) and with the human malarias P. falciparum (30–32) and P. vivax (33). The range of variation detected in the rodent malarias was very large compared with the slight variation found between the human malarias. Figure 2.5 shows how the electrophoresis gels used for enzyme typing are read and what they mean.

Studies with P. falciparum isolates found that the enzyme glucose phosphate isomerase (GPI) has two enzyme types, GPI-1 and GPI-2. Of isolates tested from patients in Africa and Asia, 25% were mixed infections, that is, these patients carried both GPI-1 and GPI-2 parasite types simultaneously; only 7% of isolates from Brazilian patients were mixed. For another enzyme, adenosine deaminase (ADA), mixed infections of ADA-1 and ADA-2 types simultaneously were again found mostly in Africa (30% of the isolates tested), while in Asia and Brazil the proportions were smaller (1.5% and 4.5%, respectively). For lactate dehydrogenase (LDH), parasites with type 1 and those with type 2 of the enzyme were found in mixed populations in 20% of the African isolates tested. However, so far only type LDH-1 parasites have been detected from Asia and Brazil.

Studies with enzyme typing of parasites have allowed the comparison of isolates of P. falciparum at two different levels: geographically, with large numbers of isolates tested and classified according to their enzyme type, and at the more restricted level of a single patient, where mixed populations of parasites can be detected in each isolate. It should be borne in mind that enzyme types, like most markers studied so far, are not necessarily related to other markers, for example, drug resistance. However, it is important to emphasize that these results cannot be generalized, since each patient represents a distinct situation. For example, in a study of an isolate from a patient that eventually exhibited resistance to treatment with mefloquine (34, 35), a mixture of parasites types GPI-1 and GPI-2 was seen. Cloning of these parasites, separated by the limited dilution technique (13), resulted in five clones, of which one was type GPI-1 and four were type GPI-2. But all the resistant parasites obtained from this patient (that is, those obtained after treatment) were type 1 only. Hence, in this particular case, resistance to mefloquine was associated with enzyme type.

Protein analysis by means of two-dimensional protein screening (36, 37) using radio-labeled parasites has also been employed to characterize different parasite populations. Proteins are separated according to their molecular weights and isoelectric points. This technique revealed the diversity among blood-stage P. falciparum. Over 100 proteins can be detected, of which 14 (designated A to N) showed differences on the gel in either weight or charge. These variant positions for each protein were numbered (for protein A, for example, A.1, A.2, etc.). Each clone from an isolate exhibits only one protein type. The variant forms of each protein are most probably due to allelic variation in the genes that code for them. Blood-stage parasites are haploid; therefore, clones possess one allele of each gene that codes for a protein in the phenotype. This research method is technically difficult, but is highly reproducible and the parasite clones stable—that is, repeated assays with the same clone population, maintained in vitro, gave the same results. Some of the protein spots detected (or lacking) cannot yet be associated with other markers, but some researchers (37) consider that protein "A" is most probably a polymorphic schizont antigen, and protein "B" a soluble antigen. The above-cited work demonstrates the genetic heterogeneity that exists in the parasite population within an isolate. This technique, better than enzyme analysis, offers a broad biochemical description of the parasite population and has also allowed confirmation that clones (obtained by means of the limited dilution technique) are indeed clones.

Some antigens have also been used for classification of parasites. The polyspecific nature of immune serum makes results obtained with this material difficult to interpret, but the production of monoclonal antibodies (which react with single epitopes) has greatly improved knowledge of antigenic diversity in parasites.

Soluble antigens are detectable in the culture media in which *P. falciparum* are maintained *in vitro*, as well as in the sera of patients who have suffered malaria attacks (38). Immunodiffusion techniques have made it possible to differentiate isolates of different geographic origin, and the presence of different antigenic types, presumably corresponding to different clones, has also been shown in individual patients (39).

Various studies (40–42) have used a number of monoclonal antibodies that bind with a high–molecular weight, polymorphic surface antigen on schizonts and merozoites. The antibodies can be used to characterize strains of the parasites, and a system was devised for serologic classification based on the parasites' antigenic polymorphism. The isolates are divided into seven serotypes (groups I–VII) according to reactivity patterns observed by indirect immunofluorescence microscopy.

Just as certain enzyme types were not found in certain geographic regions (for example, LDH-2 in Brazil), some serotypes are also lacking. Serotype group V has not yet been found in isolates from Brazil. On the other hand, using some of the techniques here described, one study identified seven different parasite populations (clones) growing simultaneously in a single patient (43).

Recently, 37 monoclonal antibody reagents, produced by different laboratories, which react against the asexual blood stage of *P. falciparum* have been analyzed and grouped according to their indirect immunofluorescence pattern (44). Antigens that show a high level of diversity and variation are of little use as potential vaccine candidates, since antigens to be used for that purpose must be consistently recognized and identified in parasites of the same species from various countries and origins and must be stable over time. Antigenic variation in *P. falciparum* was demonstrated during an infection in monkeys (12), but it was not established whether the new variants were induced by immunity or whether immune pressure only selected preexisting variants from the population.

Pulsed field gel electrophoresis, which has been used for separation of DNA molecules (chromosomes) (45–47), also allows for the differentiation of parasites and clones. Recently, bands representing 14 chromosomes from the blood-stage forms of *P. falciparum* have been purified. The understanding of malaria genetics will be greatly increased by this technique, particularly in association with hybridization methods that can identify specific genes or gene linkages.

APPLICATION IN THE FIELD

This chapter summarizes some of the research carried out with blood stages of *P. falciparum* malaria parasites. It is clear that although diagnosis of malaria is not difficult, great diversity exists among parasites in a single species, and the different types need to be properly identified.

In order to link clinical interests and the techniques described above, it is useful to discuss results obtained in some *in vivo* field tests for chloroquine susceptibility of *P. falciparum* (7). These tests, carried out when the clinical condition of the patient allows, define four types of responses: the sensitive response (S), when blood tested is negative for parasites after a standard treatment and they do not reappear; resistance type I, when asexual parasites reappear within four weeks after treatment began; type II, when there is marked reduction but no disappearance of parasitemia after treatment; and type III, when there is either no marked reduction of parasitemia following treatment or an increase. This is an important test; however, the same response may not indicate comparable parasite populations in two different patients, since the proportions of resistant-versus-sensitive parasites may be very different. Type I resistance (RI), although suggesting that the patient carried almost all sensitive parasites, also indicates that the patient carried some resistant ones that, due to their low numbers, took longer to detect. If these resistant types were transmitted to another patient, they might produce a resistance-type III (RIII) infection. It is both the number of parasites and their level of resistance that determine the time required for the infection to reappear in the patient. Therefore, an S-type response within only seven days may be misleading. Continuous and indiscriminate drug use in an area could increase the number of patients with type RIII infection, owing to selection of more resistant parasites. These studies suggest that health care institutions need to develop a very careful policy on use of antimalarial drugs, whether for prophylaxis or for treatment, since selection for resistant parasites can be initiated by the drug itself if it is not given in a proper curative dose.

OTHER HUMAN MALARIA SPECIES

Unfortunately, very little work has been done on identification of the other species of malaria parasites by the methods described above. Several authors have reported culturing *P. vivax* (48–50), but other research workers using the same methodology have been unsuccessful. Enzyme studies showed that GPI enzyme types differed from *P. falciparum* (33).

There are various theories to explain the biology of relapses caused by the relapsing plasmodia (51, 52); it is known that different strains have different relapse patterns (52). Therefore, it is believed that their diversity will be as marked as that found in *P. falciparum*.

CONCLUSION

This chapter has reviewed some of the data obtained with *P. falciparum* that show how diverse these parasites can be when isolates from different countries, or from the parasite population within one patient, are compared. These results suggest the need to continually review policy regarding the appropriate use of antimalarial drugs. It is essential that new drugs be tested in the laboratory with cloned lines of parasites of different origins in order to evaluate their *in vitro* effectiveness and to prepare for tests of their efficacy and toxicity in animal models and of their *in vivo* effectiveness and tolerance, as determined from *in vivo* clinical tests in humans.

REFERENCES

(1) Garnham, P. C. C. *Malaria Parasites and Other Haemosporidia.* Oxford: Blackwell Scientific Publications, 1966.

(2) Garnham, P. C. C. Malaria in its various vertebrate hosts. *In: Malaria*, Vol. I, Chapter 2. New York: Academic Press, 1980.

(3) Lepes, T. Technical problems related to biological characterization of malaria, as encountered in malaria control/eradication. WHO/MAL 81.934:1–7, 1981.

(4) Bruce-Chwatt, L. J. DNA probes for malaria diagnosis. *Lancet* 7:795, 1984.

(5) Post, R. J., and J. M. Crampton. Probing the unknown. *Parasitol Today* 3:380–383, 1987.

(6) Wernsdorfer, W. H., and R. L. Kouztnetsov. Drug-resistant malaria—occurrence, control and surveillance. *Bull WHO* 58(3):341–352, 1980.

(7) Peters, W. Chemotherapy of malaria. *In: Malaria*, Vol. I, Chapter 2. New York: Academic Press, 1980.

(8) World Health Organization. *Advances in Malaria Chemotherapy. Report of a WHO Scientific Group.* Technical Report Series 711. Geneva, 1984.

(9) Nelson, G. S. Problems in the identification of parasites and their vectors in relation to disease control. *In: New Approaches to the Identification of Parasites and their Vectors.* UNDP/World Bank/WHO Tropical Diseases Research Series 5, 1984.

(10) Trager, W., and J. B. Jensen. Human malaria parasites in continuous culture. *Science* 193:673–675, 1976.

(11) Hommel, M. Antigenic variation in malaria parasites. *Immunol Today* 6(1):28–33, 1985.

(12) Howard, R. Malaria: antigens and host-parasite interactions. Pp. 111–165 *in*: T. W. Pearson (ed.), *Parasite Antigens—Toward New Strategies for Vaccines,* 7. New York: Marcel Dekker, Inc., 1986.

(13) do Rosario, V. E. Cloning of naturally occurring mixed infections of malaria parasites. *Science* 212:1037–1038, 1981.

(14) Trager, W., M. Tershakovec, L. Lyandvert, H. Standley, N. Lanners, and E. Gubert. Clones of the malaria parasite *Plasmodium falciparum* obtained by microscopic selection: Their characterization with regard to knobs, chloroquine sensitivity, and formation of gametocytes. *Proc Natl Acad Sci USA* 78(10):6527–6530, 1981.

(15) Miller, L. H., S. J. Mason, J. A. Dvorak, M. H. McGiniss, and I. K. Rothman. Erythrocyte receptors for *(Plasmodium knowlesi)* malaria: Duffy blood group determinants. *Science* 189:561–563, 1975.

(16) López Antuñano, F. J., and T. T. Palmer. Sensitivity of Duffy negative erythrocytes in *Aotus* monkeys to *Plasmodium vivax* (letter). *Trans R Soc Trop Med Hyg* 72(3):319, 1978.

(17) Pasvol, G., and R. J. M. Wilson. The interaction of malaria parasites with red blood cells. *Br Med Bull* 38(2):133–140, 1982.

(18) Luzzato, L., E. A. Usanga, and G. Modiano. Genetic resistance to *Plasmodium falciparum*: Studies in the field and in cultures *in vitro*. *In: Ecology and Genetics of Host-Parasite Interaction.* London: Academic Press, 1985.

(19) Hermentin, P. Malaria invasion of human erythrocytes. *Parasitol Today* 3(2):52–55, 1987.

(20) Jensen, J. B., S. L. Hoffman, M. T. Boland, M. A. S. Akood, L. W. Laughlin, L. Kurniawan, and H. A. Marwoto. Comparison of immunity to malaria in Sudan and Indonesia: Crisis-form versus merozoite-invasion inhibition. *Proc Natl Acad Sci USA* 81:922–925, 1984.

(21) Wellems, T. E., D. Walliker, C. L. Smith, V. E. do Rosario, L. W. Maloy, R. J. Howard, R. Carter, and T. F. McCutchan. A histidine-rich protein gene marks a linkage group favored strongly in a genetic cross of *Plasmodium falciparum*. *Cell* 49:633–642, 1987.

(22) Carter, R., and L. H. Miller. Evidence for environmental modulation of gametocytogenesis in *Plasmodium falciparum* in continuous culture. *Bull WHO* 57(suppl. 1):37–52, 1979.

(23) Burkot, T. R., J. L. Williams, and I. Schneider. Infectivity to mosquitoes of *Plasmodium falciparum* clones grown *in vitro* from the same isolate. *Trans R Soc Trop Med Hyg* 78:339–341, 1984.

(24) Andre, R. G. Comparison of the susceptibility of certain Thai *Anopheles* for human malaria. Conference on Malaria Research, Pattaya, Thailand, 25–27 April 1983. Abstract.

(25) de Arruda, M., M. B. Carvalho, R. S. Nussenzweig, M. Maracic, A. W. Ferreira, and A. H. Cochrane. Potential vectors of malaria and their different susceptibility to *Plasmodium falciparum* and *Plasmodium vivax* in Northern Brazil, identified by immunoassay. *Am J Trop Med Hyg* 35(5):873–881, 1986.

(26) Sinden, R. E. The cell biology of sexual development in *Plasmodium*. *Parasitology* 86:7–28, 1983.

(27) Sinden, R. E. Sexual development of malarial parasites. *Adv Parasitol* 23:154–216, 1983.

(28) Inselburg, J. Gametocyte formation by the progeny of single *Plasmodium falciparum* schizonts. *J Parasitol* 69(3):584–591, 1983.

(29) Carter, R. Studies on enzyme variation in the murine malaria parasite *Plasmodium berghei*, *P. yoelii*, *P. vinckei* and *P. chabaudi* by starch gel electrophoresis. *Parasitology* 76:241–267, 1978.

(30) Carter, R., and I. A. McGregor. Enzyme variation in *Plasmodium falciparum* in the Gambia. *Trans R Soc Trop Med Hyg* 67:830–837, 1973.

(31) Thaithong, S., T. Sueblinwong, and G. H. Beale. Enzyme typing of some isolates of *Plasmodium falciparum* from Thailand. *Trans R Soc Trop Med Hyg* 75:268–270, 1981.

(32) Couto, A., V. do Rosario, and D. Walliker. Análise enzimática de 56 amostras de *Plasmodium falciparum* de Bacia Amazônica (Brasil). *Rev Bras Malariol Doenças Trop* 35:11–19, 1983.

(33) Mynt-Oo. Isoenzyme variation in schizonts of *P. vivax* from Burma. *Trans R Soc Trop Med Hyg* 80:1–4, 1986.

(34) Webster. H. K., S. Thaithong, K. Pavanand, K. Yongvanitchit, C. Pinswasdi, and E. F. Boudreau. Cloning of mefloquine-resistant *Plasmodium falciparum* from Thailand. WHO/MAL/84.1015:1–7, 1984.

(35) Webster, H. K., S. Thaithong, K. Pavanand, K. Yongvanitchit, C. Pinswasdi, and E. F. Boudreau. Cloning and characterization of mefloquine-resistant *Plasmodium falciparum* from Thailand. *Am J Trop Med Hyg* 34(6):1022–1027, 1985.

(36) Tait, A. Analysis of protein variation in *Plasmodium falciparum* by two-dimensional gel electrophoresis. *Mol Biochem Parasitol* 2:205–218, 1981.

(37) Fenton, B., A. Walker, and D. Walliker. Protein variation in clones of *Plasmodium falciparum* detected by two-dimensional electrophoresis. *Mol Biochem Parasitol* 16:163–183, 1985.

(38) Wilson, R. J. Serotyping *Plasmodium falciparum* malaria with S-antigens. *Nature* 284:451–452, 1980.

(39) Schoefield, L., S. Tharavanij, A. Saul, V. do Rosario, and C. Kidson. A specific S-antigen of *Plasmodium falciparum* is expressed in a proportion of primary isolates in Brazil, Thailand and Papua New Guinea. *Trans R Soc Trop Med Hyg* 79(4):493–494, 1985.

(40) Hall, R., J. S. McBride, G. Morgan, A. Tait, J. W. Zolg, D. Walliker, and J. Scaife. Antigens of the erythrocyte stages of the human malaria parasite *Plasmodium falciparum* detected by monoclonal antibodies. *Mol Biochem Parasitol* 7:247–265, 1983.

(41) McBride, J. S., D. Walliker, and G. Morgan. Antigenic diversity in the human malaria parasite *Plasmodium falciparum*. *Science* 217:254–257, 1982.

(42) McBride, J. S., C. I. Newbold, and R. Anand. Polymorphism of a high molecular weight schizont antigen of the human malaria parasite *Plasmodium falciparum*. *J Exp Med* 161:160–180, 1985.

(43) Thaithong, S., G. H. Beale, B. Fenton, J. S. McBride, V. do Rosario, A. Walker, and D. Walliker. Clonal diversity in a single isolate of the human malaria parasite *Plasmodium falciparum*. *Trans R Soc Trop Med Hyg* 78:242–245, 1984.

(44) Dayal, R., C. Decrind, and P. H. Lambert. Comparison of asexual blood-stage antigens of *Plasmodium falciparum* recognized by antibody reagents from nine laboratories. *Bull WHO* 64(3):403–414, 1986.

(45) Kemp, D. J., L. M. Corcoran, R. L. Coppel, H. D. Stahl, A. E. Bianco, G. V. Brown, and R. F. Anders. Size variation in chromosomes from independent cultured isolates of *Plasmodium falciparum*. *Nature* 315:347–350, 1985.

(46) Van der Ploeg, L. H. T., M. Smits, T. Ponnudurai, A. Vermeulen, J. H. Meuwissen, and G. Langsley. Chromosome-sized DNA molecules of *Plasmodium falciparum*. *Science* 229:658–661, 1985.

(47) Dawkins, H. J. S. Molecular weight separation of very large DNA. *Parasitol Today* 3(2):60–62, 1978.

(48) Larrouy, G., J. F. Magnaval, and F. Moro. A propos de l'obtention par culture *in vitro* de formes intra-erythrocitaires de *Plasmodium vivax*. *C R Acad Sci* (Paris) 292:929–930, 1981.

(49) Renaparkur, D. M., D. M. Pradhan, N. K. Sutar, M. V. N. Shirodkar, K. D. Sharma, V. S. Ajgaonkar, and S. N. Marathe. The continuous *in vitro* cultivation of *Plasmodium vivax*. *Physiology* 11:7–8, 1983.

(50) Brockelmann, C. R., P. Tan-Arya, and R. Laovanitch. Observation on complete schizogony of *Plasmodium vivax in vitro*. *J Protozool* 32(1):76–80, 1985.

(51) Short, H. E., and P. C. C. Garnham. Demonstration of a persisting exo-erythrocytic cycle in *P. cynomolgi* and its bearing on the production of relapses. *Br Med J* 1:1225–1228, 1948.

(52) Schmidt, L. H. Compatibility of relapse patterns of *Plasmodium cynomolgi* infections in *Rhesus* monkeys with continuous cyclical development and hypnozoite concepts of relapse. *Am J Trop Med Hyg* 36(6):1077–1099, 1986.

Chapter 3

DEVELOPMENT OF THE MALARIA PARASITE IN THE MOSQUITO: THE SPOROGONIC CYCLE

Robert W. Gwadz

The phases of the life cycle of the malaria parasite that occur in the mosquito represent a complex series of events. Because sexual, or sporogonic, reproduction of these protozoa takes place in the midgut of the mosquito vector, by convention the mosquito is considered the definitive host of the parasite, while a vertebrate, which may be man, acts as the intermediate host in which asexual, or schizogonic, reproduction occurs. Although our primary interest is the sporogonic development of the malaria parasites that infect humans—*Plasmodium falciparum*, *P. vivax*, *P. ovale*, and *P. malariae*—much of what we know about sporogonic development is based on studies of the plasmodia of birds, rodents, and nonhuman primates.

The sporogonic cycle of malaria has received increased attention in the last few years. Malaria control programs directed against the mosquito vector remain the most effective means of limiting this disease. However, vector control strategies to reduce mosquito populations, modify man/mosquito contact, or affect vector competence have all come under review in response to the double threat of insecticide resistance in the mosquito and drug resistance in the parasite. At the same time, the development of two of the most important malaria vaccine candidates—the infection-blocking sporozoite vaccine and the transmission-blocking gamete vaccine—has depended heavily on utilizing stages of the parasite that grow in the mosquito. This awareness of the importance of the sporogonic stages and their mosquito hosts has prompted a series of research efforts. It is anticipated that a better understanding of the sporogonic stages and their development in the mosquito will lead to the evolution of more effective strategies for the control of malaria, one of the world's most feared vector-borne diseases.

PHASES OF DEVELOPMENT IN THE MOSQUITO

THE BLOOD MEAL

Mosquitoes feed on water, nectars and sugar solutions, or blood. Only female mosquitoes will seek a blood meal, which they need as a protein source for egg production, and it is in the course of blood feeding that the protozoan parasite of malaria, as well as a wide range of other pathogenic organisms, is initially ingested and later transmitted.

Mosquitoes are attracted by odors emanating from the vertebrate host; blood feeding behavior is initiated in response to host body heat and further motivated by phagostimulants present in the blood. A number of culicine mosquitoes, including *Aedes aegypti, Culex pipiens,* and *Culiseta inornata,* have been shown to respond to adenosine triphosphate (ATP) in the blood as a phagostimulant. However, similar studies with four anopheline species (*Anopheles freeborni, An. stephensi, An. dirus,* and *An. gambiae*) demonstrated no requirement for blood ATP to induce ingestion *(1).* When a mosquito feeds, the blood meal is normally shunted to the midgut, while sugar meals are held in the ventral diverticulum *(2).* The quantity of blood imbibed during feeding is under nervous control *(3)* and can be affected by prior ingestion of sugar meals or the presence of mature eggs in the ovaries. Some anophelines, for example, *An. stephensi,* may imbibe up to 10 μl, retain 2 μl of packed erythrocytes, and excrete the excess as a bright red, almost erythrocyte-free rectal fluid (Figure 3.1) *(4).* In other anopheline species, there is little or no excretion during the feeding process.

The midgut epithelial cells start to synthesize digestive enzymes soon after the blood meal, with peak enzyme activity at 24 hours after feeding. Once the blood is digested and nutrients absorbed, the residue, undigested erythrocytes, and digestive enzymes are voided. Concurrent with digestion, oogenesis is initiated and oocytes mature. Two or three days after the blood meal, a fertilized female will deposit her eggs at an appropriate site and prepare to feed again. This cycle of blood meal and oviposition, followed by another blood meal, is maintained throughout the life of the female mosquito. It requires repeated contacts with the vertebrate host, allows time for multiplication or maturation of parasites and pathogens within the mosquito, and permits eventual infection of other individual hosts during subsequent feedings.

SEXUAL STAGES OF THE MALARIA PARASITE IN THE VERTEBRATE HOST

The malaria parasite undergoes asexual multiplication within erythrocytes of the vertebrate host by the process of schizogony, which produces merozoites that eventually lyse the infected cells and invade other erythrocytes. This asexual cycle of erythrocyte invasion, multiplication, rupture, and reinvasion is associated with the complex pathology of the malaria infection. At the same time, certain merozoites develop into sexual forms, the male and female gametocytes. Although the process of gametocytogenesis in the vertebrate host is poorly understood, *in vitro* studies have described factors that can affect it *(5–7).*

In some malarias, for example, those caused by *P. vivax, P. cynomolgi, P. knowlesi, P. berghei,* and *P. gallinaceum,* gametocytes appear at patency simultaneously with the first asexual parasites detectable in the blood. On the other hand, in *P. falciparum* malaria, the appearance of mature gametocytes in blood is delayed by about two weeks after the beginning of the erythrocytic cycle, reflecting the slow maturation of gametocytes in this parasite and sequestration of the immature stages *(8).*

Malaria has long been distinguished from other fevers by the intermittent but highly regular nature of its chills and fever. Malaria caused by *P. vivax* and *P. falciparum* was described as tertian, with fever every other day (a 48-hour cycle of development), and *P. malariae* malaria was termed quartan because of its 72-hour cycle. It has been suggested that this synchronicity evolved as a mechanism to assure the presence of mature gametocytes at the time when the nocturnal anopheline mosquito vectors come to feed (9). The "Hawking phenomenon," so named after its describer, is demonstrated by the simian parasites *P. knowlesi*, *P. cynomolgi*, and *P. coatneyi* (10). In these species, gametocytes are infectious to mosquitoes for a relatively short time period (6-10 hours) coinciding with the evening hours when the anopheline vectors are feeding, but lose their infectivity during the day when the vectors are absent. However, the phenomenon is not universal; *P. falciparum* gametocytes are both long-lived (half-life of 2.5 days) and infectious to mosquitoes at all hours (11).

Factors controlling the capacity of gametocytes of the various malarias to infect mosquitoes are poorly understood. It has been shown that repeated passage by injection of infected blood can result in the loss of gametocyte production, for example, in *P. berghei* of rodents and *P. lophurae* of ducks. However, syringe passage of *P. cynomolgi* and *P. knowlesi* in monkeys over several decades caused no reduction in either gametocyte production or infectivity to mosquitoes (12).

Infectivity of gametocytes to mosquitoes can be affected by host immunity or the relationship of gametocytemia to the level of asexual parasitemia. The gametocytes of *P. vivax*, *P. cynomolgi*, and *P. knowlesi* are most infectious during the early stages of a primary attack or recrudescence. Infectivity of circulating gametocytes to mosquitoes is significantly reduced on the day of peak asexual parasitemia and may fail completely as that parasitemia wanes (8). In contrast, infectious gametocytes of *P. falciparum* may persist in the circulation for weeks at a time.

SEXUAL STAGES OF THE MALARIA PARASITE IN THE MOSQUITO

SPOROGONIC CYCLE

In the transmission of malaria, mosquitoes become infected when they ingest a vertebrate host's blood containing mature gametocytes. In the mosquito midgut, macrogametocytes (female) and microgametocytes (male) shed the red cell membranes that surround them and develop into gametes. Microgametogenesis is a particularly dramatic event, wherein a single microgametocyte gives rise to eight sperm-like, highly vigorous flagellated microgametes (Figure 3.2). Exflagellation can be seen readily in infected blood, and it was this process observed in the blood of a French soldier in Algeria that led Laveran in 1880 to definitively associate parasitized erythrocytes with malarial disease.

Although most plasmodia will exflagellate *in vitro* under optimal conditions, exflagellation *in vivo* is stimulated by a factor or factors present in the mosquito midgut (13–15). Species-specific stimulation of exflagellation is but one of many mechanisms that determine if a mosquito can act as host to a malaria parasite. The avian parasite, *P. elongatum*, will exflagellate only in the midgut of its natural vector *C. quinquefasciatus*, and not in *Aedes* or *Anopheles* mosquitoes; a *Culex*-specific factor in the midgut appears to be necessary (16). Similarly, the monkey malaria *P. cynomolgi*, which is normally transmitted by anopheline mosquitoes, fails to exflagellate in the gut of *C. thalassius* or to compete fertilization in *Ae. aegypti* (17). Structural changes of the macro- and microgametocytes during gametogenesis have been described by a number of authors and reviewed elsewhere (18).

The sporogonic cycle begins in the mosquito midgut minutes after the blood meal. Fertilization is probably accomplished within the first 20-30 minutes (19), during which time the macrogametocytes mature into macrogametes and each one accepts a microgamete to become a zygote. The zygote then elongates, first to a banana-shaped form and later to the vermiform ookinete (Figure 3.2) (20).

Development of the malaria parasite within the mosquito's midgut and ookinete invasion of the midgut epithelium appear to require erythrocyte factors released during digestion of the blood meal (21). However, once beyond the epithelial barrier, those factors are not essential for parasite survival. Ookinetes injected directly into the hemocoel will develop in both female and male mosquitoes in the absence of erythrocyte factors (22).

The ookinete penetrates the midgut epithelium either through or between the epithelial cells and settles beneath the basal lamina of the outer gut wall (Figure 3.2). Penetration of the gut is completed within 24 hours after the blood meal, and oocyst development commences thereafter. Ultrastructural studies of oocyst development and sporozoite formation have been performed on a number of rodent, avian, and monkey plasmodia. A detailed study of the sporogonic development of P. falciparum revealed that oocysts are of uniform size in low-density infections, but may vary widely in size when the infection is intense (23). The length of time required to go from ookinete to mature sporozoite depends on the species of malaria parasite, the species of mosquito host, the ambient temperature, and the density of infection. Likewise, the time required for an oocyst to reach its maximum volume and full maturation varies with different species of anophelines, the temperature of the microclimate, and the intensity of infection. Also, two mosquito species feeding on the same host can support significantly different numbers of oocysts (24). It is important to note that most infected vector mosquitoes captured in the field have very low oocyst counts; the majority have a single oocyst on the gut membrane, and the remainder usually have five or fewer (25, 26).

It had been generally assumed that the rupture of ripe oocysts and release of mature sporozoites into the hemocoel of the mosquito was a single dramatic event. However, scanning electron microscopic studies have shown that oocysts do not rupture, but rather that sporozoites escape gradually through the oocyst wall by way of small perforations that may become enlarged as emergence progresses (Figure 3.2) (27).

Once free in the hemolymph of its mosquito host, the sporozoite must find its way to the salivary glands. Only from there can the sporozoite be transferred to a vertebrate when the mosquito next feeds (Figure 3.2). It is not clear if sporozoites actively seek the salivary glands or are carried randomly through the hemocoel until they contact the glands. However, a mechanism by which the sporozoites recognize the salivary glands appears to exist. Supporting this notion are experiments showing that P. knowlesi developing in An. freeborni produced sporozoites that could not invade that mosquito species' salivary glands. However, when salivary glands from An. dirus, a natural vector of P. knowlesi, were implanted into infected An. freeborni, those glands were invaded by sporozoites. A specific membrane receptor appears to be necessary to facilitate sporozoite invasion of salivary glands (28).

The sporozoite undergoes significant changes during its journey from the oocyst to residence in the salivary glands. Oocyst sporozoites are weakly infectious or completely noninfectious to the vertebrate host, are weakly immunogenic as compared to salivary gland sporozoites, and react weakly to antisporozoite-specific immune serum, giving little or no circumsporozoitic reaction. They also show markedly different patterns of motility as compared to salivary gland sporozoites (29).

When it contacts the salivary gland (Figure 3.3), the sporozoite must penetrate the basal membrane, pass intracellularly through a secretory cell to a central canal of the salivary gland, and eventually move into the salivary duct (30). When the mosquito feeds, salivary fluids that prevent clotting during feeding are injected into the wound made by its mouthparts. This injection carries sporozoites, which infect the vertebrate host, reinitiating the cycle.

The number of sporozoites in the salivary glands of an infected mosquito is usually directly related to the number of oocysts that developed on the mosquito's gut. Heavier gut infections give rise to heavier gland infections. It has been estimated that a single oocyst of P. *falciparum* may produce approximately 10,000 sporozoites (31), but not all of these will reach the salivary glands. Heavy gut infections, unusual in nature, may produce gland infections in excess of 300,000 sporozoites per mosquito (Figure 3.4).

Although a single sporozoite is capable of initiating infection in the vertebrate host, the precise number of sporozoites injected by a feeding mosquito is unknown. However, the number of sporozoites in the salivary gland directly determines the number of sporozoites available for injection.

FACTORS GOVERNING THE SUSCEPTIBILITY AND VECTOR COMPETENCE OF MOSQUITOES

Of the thousands of mosquito species, only a relatively small number are involved in the transmission of malaria to humans. The factors that regulate vector susceptibility are numerous, complex, and poorly understood. Only mosquitoes of the genus *Anopheles* transmit the plasmodia that produce malaria in humans. However, to be a good vector of human malaria, the anopheline mosquito must show a tendency to bite man (anthropophily), live long enough for the parasite to develop, and provide the appropriate physiological environment to support the development of the malaria parasite. The mosquito's ability to act as an efficient host for the developing parasite and support the sporogonic development of any species of *Plasmodium* is under genetic control (32). Manipulation of the genes that regulate susceptibility in mosquitoes has been suggested as an alternative method for malaria control. The replacement of natural vector populations with populations of the same species genetically refractory to parasite development could prevent normal transmission of the parasite. Some genetic manipulations of this sort have been described and others are being developed (Figure 3.5) (33, 34). However, it is important to note that even if they prove feasible, such schemes for population replacement may not be available for decades and may be applicable only under very specific conditions.

The concept of immunization with malaria antigens derived from gametes has received considerable attention. Transmission-blocking immunity induced in the human host with such antigens would affect the sporogonic development of the malaria parasite by interrupting the sexual cycle within the mosquito (35–38). After immunization with gamete antigens, an individual could contract malaria and produce gametocytes. However, when a feeding mosquito imbibed gametocytes plus anti-gamete antibodies in the blood meal, fertilization of the malaria parasite would be blocked, ookinetes would not be formed, and the infection in the mosquito would be aborted.

Transmission-blocking immunization schemes would affect the epidemiology of malaria in two important ways:

(1) An immunized individual could not act as a reservoir of infection and would serve only as a dead-end for the parasite.

(2) When used in combination with antigens directed against the sporozoite or asexual stages of the malaria parasite, transmission-blocking antigens could prevent the transmission of any variant forms of the parasite that might arise. Variant or mutant parasite strains could pose a significant threat to any broadly applied malaria immunization program, and blockage of their transmission could ensure the success of the campaign.

It must be emphasized that the various malaria vaccine candidates, whether directed against sporozoites or asexual stages or the sexual stages in the mosquito, although showing great promise, may be years away from application in the field.

Studies of the sporogonic cycle of plasmodia have been important in clarifying the epidemiology of malaria by providing efficient tools for determining sporozoite rates in infected mosquitoes in the field. Further research on the sporogonic development of plasmodia in mosquitoes should yield important new methods for controlling malaria.

REFERENCES

(1) Galun, R., L. C. Koontz, R. W. Gwadz, and J. P. M. Ribeiro. Effect of ATP analogues on the gorging response of *Aedes aegypti*. *Physiol Entomol* 10:275–281, 1985.

(2) Trembly, H. L. The distribution of certain liquids in the esophageal diverticula and stomach of mosquitoes. *Am J Trop Med Hyg* 1:693–710, 1952.

(3) Gwadz, R. W. Regulation of blood meal size in the mosquito. *J Insect Physiol* 15:2039–2044, 1969.

(4) Briegel, H., and L. Rezzonico. Concentration of host blood protein during feeding by anopheline mosquitoes (Diptera: Culicidae). *J Med Entomol* 22:612–618, 1985.

(5) Smalley, M. E. *Plasmodium falciparum* gametocytogenesis *in vitro*. *Nature* 264:271–272, 1976.

(6) Carter, R., and L. H. Miller. Evidence for environmental modulation of gametocytogenesis in *Plasmodium falciparum* in continuous culture. *Bull WHO* 57(Suppl. 1):37–52, 1979.

(7) Inselburg, J. Gametocyte formation by the progeny of single *Plasmodium falciparum* schizonts. *J Parasitol* 69:584–591, 1983.

(8) Carter, R., and R. W. Gwadz. Infectiousness and gamete immunization in malaria. Pp. 263–297 *in:* J. P. Kreser (ed.), *Malaria*, Vol. 3. New York: Academic Press, 1980.

(9) Hawking, F., M. J. Worms, and K. Gammage. 24- and 48-hour cycles of malaria parasites in the blood; their purpose, production and control. *Trans R Soc Trop Med Hyg* 62:731–760, 1968.

(10) Garnham, P. C. C., and K. G. Powers. Periodicity of infectivity of plasmodial gametocytes: The "Hawking phenomenon." *Int J Parasitol* 4:103–106, 1974.

(11) Smalley, M. E., and R. E. Sinden. *Plasmodium falciparum* gametocytes: Their longevity and infectivity. *Parasitology* 74:1–8, 1977.

(12) Vanderberg, J. P., and R. W. Gwadz. The transmission by mosquitoes of plasmodia in the laboratory. Pp. 153–234 *in:* J. P. Kreier (ed.), *Malaria*, Vol. 2. New York: Academic Press, 1980.

(13) Carter, R., and M. M. Nijhout. Control of gamete formation (exflagellation) in malaria parasites. *Science* 195:407–409, 1977.

(14) Nijhout, M. M., and R. Carter. Gamete development in malaria parasites: Bicarbonate-dependent stimulation by pH *in vitro*. *Parasitology* 76:39–53, 1978.

(15) Nijhout, M. M. *Plasmodium gallinaceum*: Exflagellation stimulated by a mosquito factor. *Exp Parasitol* 48:75–80, 1979.

(16) Micks, D. W., P. F. De Caires, and L. B. Franco. The relationship of exflagellation in avian plasmodia to pH and immunity in the mosquito. *Am J Hyg* 48:182–190, 1948.

(17) Omar, M. S. Vergleichende Beobachtungen uber die Entwicklung von *Plasmodium cynomolgi bastianellii* in *Anopheles stephensi* und *Anopheles albimanus*. *Z Tropenmed Parasitol* 19:370–389, 1968.

(18) Sinden, R. E. Sexual development in malarial parasites. *Adv Parasitol* 22:153–216, 1983.

(19) Carter, R., R. W. Gwadz, and F. M. McAuliffe. *Plasmodium gallinaceum*: Transmission-blocking immunity in chickens. I. Comparative immunogenicity of gametocyte- and gamete-containing preparations. *Exp Parasitol* 47:185–193, 1979.

(20) Gass, R. F. The ultrastructure of cultured *Plasmodium gallinaceum* ookinetes: A comparison of intact stages with forms damaged by extracts from blood-fed, susceptible *Aedes aegypti*. *Acta Tropica* 36:323–334, 1979.

(21) Rosenberg, R., and L. C. Koontz. *Plasmodium gallinaceum*: Erythrocyte factor essential for zygote infection of *Aedes aegypti*. *Exp Parasitol* 57:158–164, 1984.

(22) Rosenberg, R. Susceptibility of a male mosquito to malaria. *J Parasitol* 70:827, 1984.

(23) Sinden, R. E., and K. Strong. An ultrastructural study of the sporogonic development of *Plasmodium falciparum* in *Anopheles gambiae*. *Trans R Soc Trop Med Hyg* 72:477–491, 1978.

(24) Coatney, G. R., W. E. Collins, McW. Warren, and P. G. Contacos. *The Primate Malarias*. Washington, D.C.: U.S. Department of Health, Education and Welfare, 1971.

(25) Collins, F. H., F. Zavala, P. M. Graves, A. H. Cochrane, R. W. Gwadz, J. Akoh, and R. S. Nussenzweig. First field trial of an immunoradiometric assay for the detection of malaria sporozoites in mosquitoes. *Am J Trop Med Hyg* 33:538–543, 1984.

(26) Pringle, G. A quantitative study of naturally acquired malaria infections in *Anopheles gambiae* and *Anopheles funestus* in a highly malarious area of East Africa. *Trans R Soc Trop Med Hyg* 60:626–632, 1966.

(27) Sinden, R. E. Excystment by sporozoites of malaria parasites. *Nature* 252:314, 1974.

(28) Rosenberg, R. Inability of *Plasmodium knowlesi* sporozoites to invade *Anopheles freeborni* salivary glands. *Am J Trop Med Hyg* 34:687–691, 1985.

(29) Vanderberg, J. P. Studies on the motility of *Plasmodium* sporozoites. *J Protozool* 21:527–537, 1974.

(30) Sterling, C. R., M. Aikawa, and J. P. Vanderberg. The passage of *Plasmodium berghei* sporozoites through the salivary glands of *Anopheles stephensi*: An electron microscope study. *J Parasitol* 59:593–605, 1973.

(31) Pringle, G. A count of the sporozoites in an oocyst of *Plasmodium falciparum*. *Trans R Soc Trop Med Hyg* 59:289–290, 1965.

(32) Curtis, C. F., and P. M. Graves. Genetic variation in the ability of insects to transmit filariae, trypanosomes, and malarial parasites. Pp. 31-62 *in*: *Current Topics in Vector Research*, Vol. 1. New York: Praeger Publishers, 1983.

(33) Kilama, W. L., and G. B. Craig, Jr. Monofactorial inheritance of susceptibility to *Plasmodium gallinaceum* in *Aedes aegypti*. *Ann Trop Med Parasitol* 63:419–432, 1969.

(34) Collins, F. H., R. K. Sakai, K. D. Vernick, S. Paskewitz, D. C. Seeley, L. H. Miller, W. E. Collins, C. Campbell, and R. W. Gwadz. Genetic selection of a *Plasmodium*-refractory strain of the malaria vector *Anopheles gambiae*. *Science* 234:607–610, 1986.

(35) Gwadz, R. W. Malaria: Successful immunizations against the sexual stages of *Plasmodium gallinaceum*. *Science* 193:1150–1151, 1976.

(36) Carter, R., and D. H. Chen. Malaria transmission blocked by immunization with gametes of the malaria parasite. *Nature* 263:57–60, 1976.

(37) Gwadz, R. W., and I. Green. Malaria immunization in rhesus monkeys. A vaccine effective against both the sexual and asexual stages of *Plasmodium knowlesi*. *J Exp Med* 148:1311–1323, 1978.

(38) Carter, R., L. H. Miller, J. Rener, D. C. Kaushal, N. Kumar, P. M. Graves, C. A. Grotendorst, R. W. Gwadz, C. French, and D. Wirth. Target antigens in malaria transmission blocking immunity. *Philos Trans R Soc Lond* (Biol) 307:201–213, 1984.

Chapter 4

CLINICAL FEATURES OF MALARIAL INFECTION[1]

Marcos Boulos

INCUBATION PERIOD

The incubation period begins when an infected mosquito inoculates sporozoites directly into the capillaries of the human host, and ends when the latter shows clinical symptoms of the disease.

For naturally contracted malaria, the incubation period varies from seven days to eight months, depending on the parasite species and strain, the number of parasites in the blood, and previous exposure to malaria. The incubation period for malaria transmitted through multiple bites from different anopheline mosquitoes may be as short as seven days in some instances. On the other hand, mainly in temperate zones, it may last up to eight months or more.

In malaria caused by *P. vivax*, the great variations in the incubation period are due to the fact that this species is polymorphous, with two kinds of sporozoites (tachysporozoites and bradysporozoites). Whether the incubation period is short or long depends on the proportion of the kinds of sporozoites injected by the mosquito (*1, 2*).

When malaria is induced by the transfusion of parasitized blood, the incubation period varies from 10 hours to 60 days, depending on the species of *Plasmodium* and the number of parasites in the inoculum. In exceptional instances, however, this period may be much shorter (*3*).

PREPATENT PERIOD

The prepatent period is associated with the malarial infection's pre-erythrocytic cycle in the human liver. This period begins when the mosquito inoculates the sporozoites and lasts until the first merozoites issuing from the hepatic schizonts invade the erythrocytes, thus beginning the erythrocytic cycle or blood schizogony.

This period varies according to the plasmodial species responsible for the infection, and this variation can be explained by the difference in the number of merozoites produced by the hepatic schizonts. It is estimated that the number of merozoites released by each schizont is 2,000 for *P. malariae*, 10,000 for *P. vivax*, 15,000 for *P. ovale*, and 40,000 for *P. falciparum*. The prepatent period only can be demonstrated by means of subinoculation of blood.

---

[1]The terminology used in this chapter follows that in *Terminology of Malaria and of Malaria Eradication*, Geneva, World Health Organization, 1963.

SUBPATENT PERIOD
(Subpatent Parasitemia)

The subpatent period covers the interval from the time when the first hepatic merozoites invade the erythrocytes until the blood merozoites invade enough erythrocytes in the bloodstream to be detectable (patent) through a routine blood test. During this period, the parasitized red blood cells are so few that they are diluted throughout the patient's bloodstream. An individual has an estimated 90 ml of blood per kg of body weight; therefore, the parasitized blood cells cannot be detected through standard microscopic examination of a minute blood sample. The subpatent period ends when there are enough infected red cells to be observed in a routine blood test.

PATENT PERIOD
(Patent Parasitemia)

The patent period usually is associated with the clinical manifestations of malaria, and coincides with the period during which the plasmodia are observed in a sample of peripheral blood. Parasites may be found in the blood of semi-immune individuals even without clinical symptoms. For example, in the endemic region of the Brazilian Amazon, 17% of the patients are asymptomatic.[2]

CLINICAL FEATURES OF AN ACUTE ATTACK

In a few patients, prodromic symptoms appear several days before the malaria paroxysms. The patient feels discomfort and experiences occasional headache, myalgia, nausea, vomiting, asthenia, fatigue, anorexia, and slight fever. These symptoms are nonspecific, since they can be observed in other communicable diseases.

An acute malaria attack is characterized by a set of febrile paroxysms which exhibit four successive stages: chills, fever, sweating, and apyrexia.

In most malaria patients, symptoms appear suddenly with a chill that can last from 15 to 60 minutes (occasionally two hours). The symptoms involve a sudden rise in body temperature with a feeling of extreme cold, a chill with intense general shivering, and teeth chattering. This may be accompanied by headache, nausea, and vomiting. The pulse is weak and rapid. The skin is dry and has pronounced wrinkles. The lips are cyanotic. At this stage, especially in children, convulsions may occur. The period of fever lasts from two to six hours and begins as the chill ends. The patient begins to feel warm, the face becomes hyperemic, the pulse is strong, and the skin is dry and hot. The headache, which generally begins in the previous stage, intensifies and the nausea and vomiting may continue. Breathing is rapid and the patient is thirsty. Body temperature may reach 40°C or more and does not respond to antipyretics. Some patients may become delirious.

The period of sweating lasts from two to four hours. The fever drops quickly and the headache, thirst, and discomfort diminish. The patient experiences relief

---

[2] Personal observation.

and calm. When the sweating ends, the patient feels tired and weak; free of symptoms, he can sleep soundly.

The paroxysm can last from 6 to 12 hours. However, one or all the phases may fail to become apparent, which can lead to a wrong diagnosis. Eruptions of labial and nasal herpes may occur.

During the initial attacks, the periods of febrile paroxysm probably will not be well defined. This continues until a population of parasites predominates and the schizogony of most of them ends cyclically and in synchronization. As long as there are several unsynchronized populations of parasites, the patient may have a continuous, subcontinuous, or remittent fever or an intermittent fever with remissions. The fever is directly related to the release of blood merozoites upon the breakup of the parasitized erythrocytes when schizogony ends. Therefore, during the first attack or attacks, the fever is generally remittent. Once the schizogony of the predominating parasite population is synchronized, the fever will become intermittent. In that instance, the paroxysms will be characteristic of tertian or quartan malaria, occurring every 48 hours in the case of infections caused by *P. falciparum*, *P. vivax*, and *P. ovale* and every 72 hours in the case of *P. malariae*.

One characteristic of malarial fever is the presence of paroxysms at specific intervals, even at the same time of the day. Following the fever is a period of apyrexia lasting approximately 42 to 60 hours. However, this characteristic only appears when the infection is caused by a single brood of parasites that end their schizogony at the same time.

Study of the clinical manifestations of 1,380 malaria cases (991 due to *P. falciparum* and 389 due to *P. vivax*) established that 96.2% of the patients experienced fever, 83.6% headache, 52.3% myalgia, 36.2% nausea or vomiting, 29.6% chills, 9.1% sweating, and 6.3% diarrhea. No differences between the two kinds of malaria were found with regard to the frequency of the clinical manifestations.[3]

ORIGIN OF SUBSEQUENT ATTACKS

If the span between two acute malaria attacks is longer than expected for the periodic paroxysms characteristic of the species of plasmodia causing the infection, a new attack is under way. If it is possible to confirm that the subsequent attack is due to other infective bites by anophelines, the attack is considered a reinfection.

In an inadequately treated malarial infection, both the patent parasitemia and the series of febrile paroxysms may recur weeks or months after the original attack. Thus, there may be a period of parasitic latency during which a routine examination of the peripheral blood shows no parasites and/or a period of clinical latency during which the patient shows no signs or symptoms of the disease.

Parasitic recrudescence is the recurrence of patent parasitemia due to parasites that have remained in the blood at a density below the threshold of microscopic detection (fewer than 10 parasites per microliter of blood). When the number of parasites rises above the pyrogenic threshold, thus causing a new acute attack, this is called clinical recrudescence. It occurs after latent periods lasting from one to eight weeks.

---

[3] Personal observation.

Reinfection of the blood may be due to hepatic merozoites arising from hypnozoites. In other words, a second patent parasitemia occurs which in turn brings about a new acute attack known as a relapse. The number and frequency of relapses is associated with the species (*vivax* or *ovale*) and strain of plasmodia. Various authors have classified attacks following the first attack of the initial infection according to the length of latency. After a short interval of less than eight weeks, a subsequent attack is called a recrudescence, and after a long interval of more than 24 weeks, it is called a relapse (2–4).

Factors such as fatigue, pregnancy, coexisting diseases, and cold have been correlated to relapses, but the mechanism causing them is unknown.

There are no differences with regard to clinical signs and symptoms between the primary attacks and subsequent recrudescences or relapses. Moreover, in practice it is very difficult to distinguish between a recrudescence or relapse and a reinfection when the patient remains in an area of transmission.

Figure 4.1 shows the course of the malarial infection and indicates the difference between recrudescences and relapses.

CLINICAL FORMS

Malaria's clinical forms can be divided into light, moderate, serious, and critical. Classification depends on several factors, such as the intensity and duration of the fever and general symptoms, the level of parasitemia, and the degree of anemia (2).

The light form is related to the development of malaria in semi-immune individuals who already have had several episodes, or in individuals with a good immediate immune-system reaction. In such patients, the fever is not very high; the general symptoms, if any, are mild, and the parasitemia is low (generally below 0.1%). Although there may be anemia, it is not pronounced, and the hematocrit remains normal.

The moderate form is typical of nonimmune persons; they show the typical febrile paroxysm with periods of cold, heat, and sweating. Body temperature is high and climbs during the crisis, and the general symptoms are more intense, with severe headache. Parasitemia varies from 0.1% to 0.5%, and measures of hemoglobin level, number of red cells, and hematocrit indicate a moderate anemia.

The serious and critical forms, with few exceptions, occur in infections caused by *P. falciparum*.

The serious form occurs in nonimmune individuals, pregnant women, and children. Febrile paroxysm is uncommon. The patient runs a persistent fever which is not very high, and there are no chills or sweating. The headache is severe, vomiting is frequent, and there may be delirium. Up to 2% of the erythrocytes may be parasitized and anemia is intense, with a notable reduction in hemoglobin and hematocrit.

If the patient does not receive specific, suitable, and timely treatment, the critical form may develop. The above-mentioned signs and symptoms are more severe, and complications appear. The most frequent manifestations concern the kidneys, lungs, liver, brain, and blood. The fever varies but is frequently high, the headache and vomiting are persistent, and the urine diminishes and becomes concentrated. Icterus, intense tachypnea, petechiae, and small petechial effusions, mainly in the ocular conjunctiva, may be seen. The patient experiences confusion and sluggish reasoning. The parasitemia is more than 2% and may reach 30% or more. The anemia is very intense, and the patient may have a 50% reduction in hemoglobin after one week of illness.

DIFFERENT CLINICAL FORMS DEPENDENT UPON THE PLASMODIUM CAUSING THE INFECTION

Nonrelapsing malaria caused by *P. falciparum* (malignant tertian malaria)

In the absence of timely diagnosis and specific treatment, patients with *P. falciparum* infections stand a high risk of dying or becoming severely ill from malaria. Although short-term recrudescences may occur, there are no relapses after one to four weeks following the primary attack.

In Africa this is the most common of all malarias. On other continents a high incidence may occur in tropical areas. Due to the large number of merozoites released from the hepatic schizonts and to the fact that the parasites invade erythrocytes of every age, *P. falciparum* malaria has a shorter incubation period than other human malarias. The febrile paroxysms are not as well defined, especially among individuals infected for the first time. If it is not appropriately diagnosed and treated on time, complicated and serious forms may develop.

The incubation period is from 7 to 14 days and is shorter in the high endemicity areas in which *P. falciparum* resistant to anti-malarial drugs proliferates.

The disease begins with fever of variable intensity, headache, back and leg pains, prostration, anorexia, nausea, vomiting, and occasional diarrhea.

The fever may be continuous, irregular, or intermittent. An intermittent paroxysmal tertian fever more often appears in residents of endemic regions having a certain degree of immunity. The continuous and irregular fever generally occurs at the beginning of the infection and is related to the asynchronic development of different parasite populations in the red blood cells.

As the disease progresses, the symptoms become more severe, with the appearance of confusion and anxiety. The fever, which is irregular or continuous, may surpass 40°C. Convulsions may occur, especially in children. The tachycardia and tachypnea become more intense, indicating a possible pulmonary complication. The spleen and liver are generally palpable and painful. Icterus and signs of hemorrhage may appear at a subsequent stage. Figures 4.2 to 4.4 show different types of febrile curves in patients infected with *P. falciparum*.

Several factors determine the severity of development of malaria caused by *P. falciparum*: previous experience with malaria, the quantity and strain of the plasmodia inoculated, and, above all, the timeliness with which suitable treatment is begun.

In a small-scale epidemic of malaria caused by *P. falciparum* in a nonendemic region, several cases of malaria with a benign development were observed, despite the delay in diagnosing and treating them (more than 15 days). On the other hand, there were patients with high parasitemia who developed complicated forms, with changes in several organs. This took place when the initial lesions continued to develop despite the fact that the etiologic treatment eliminated the parasitemia. This phenomenon is known as the cascade syndrome (Figure 4.5) (5).

The main complications causing high parasitemias by *P. falciparum* are the following:

Cerebral malaria.   It is estimated that from 0.8% to 2% of patients with *P. falciparum* malaria exhibit brain changes *(6)*. These alterations are due to the fact that the red blood cells infected by the parasites in patients with an intense infection obstruct the cerebral capillaries. This probably occurs due to the parasitized red cells' reduced ability to change shape and to their adherence to the vascular endothelium by means of the knobs on their surfaces *(7)*.

Symptoms may begin slowly, although they are generally sudden (80% of the cases). Severe headache, hyperpyrexia, vomiting, and drowsiness appear. In children there are convulsions. The patient is affected by tachypnea and becomes comatose, with contracted pupils and with elimination or exacerbation of the deep reflexes *(6)*.

Breathing is rapid. In a final stage it becomes arrhythmic (Cheyne-Stokes respiration), with stertor caused by acute pulmonary edema, which is frequent *(6, 7)*.

Several neurologic symptoms are present, and these may simulate meningitis, intoxication, acute delirium, and epilepsy. Ocular alterations have been described, such as keratitis, uveitis, retinitis pigmentosa, optic neuritis, and paresis of the ocular muscle. Retinal hemorrhage was observed in 14.6% of the patients *(8)*. This complication is observed mainly in holoendemic regions among children younger than five years.

Sequelae such as hemiplegia, cerebellar ataxia, and deafness, although they may occur, are rare *(6)*.

Cerebral edema can lead to death. Lethality varies from 4% to 50%.

Pulmonary malaria.   Respiratory signs and symptoms occur in 3% to 10% of the patients. Clinical manifestations vary from alterations in the upper respiratory channels to acute pulmonary edema *(9)*. The symptoms may begin gradually or suddenly, with fever, cough, headache, expectoration, and vague pain. The occurrence of adventitious sound seldom can be detected in the clinical examination *(10)*.

In malaria there are several mechanisms that can lead to acute pulmonary edema. The patient develops tachypnea, with a respiratory frequency of up to 40 breaths per minute; there is a reduction in the arterial oxygen and signs of central nervous system dysfunction. A common final condition is the appearance of pulmonary edema associated with cerebral malaria caused by *P. falciparum* (Figure 4.6).

Renal lesion.   The glomerulonephritis that may exist during the development of malaria caused by *P. falciparum* is discrete and temporary. General signs and symptoms are similar to those of uncomplicated malaria, although more severe.

Most patients develop oliguria, all are anemic, and many exhibit significant hemolysis. Few show a reduction in the level of potassium in serum and most exhibit azotemia *(2)*. Almost all patients have other simultaneous complications which are generally more serious than the renal deficiency. The pathogenic mechanisms that explain the renal alterations in *P. falciparum* malaria are shown in Figure 4.7.

Hepatic changes.   All malaria cases affect the liver. Signs of hepatic alterations also appear in patients with apparently uncomplicated malaria *(11–13)*. The digestive signs observed during an acute attack of malaria are not associated with the hepatic disease, but rather are caused by the malarial paroxysm itself or by the fever *(12)*.

Hepatomegaly was observed in 57% of patients infected for the first time, and it appeared between 5 and 10 days after the disease's onset. Nevertheless, it was more severe in patients with repeated infections. This parameter is not indicative of the degree of hepatic dysfunction (14). Icterus may occur in certain uncomplicated cases, but is more severe in complicated ones.

Among the hepatic enzymes, the aminotransferases seem to be the most valuable for demonstrating hepatic lesions. When the lesions are severe, these enzymes may reach levels up to 10 times above normal (13).

Blood changes.   Anemia is one of the most important complications of malaria in children living in endemic areas, and it is the most serious cause of morbidity in adults infected by P. falciparum (15).

The merozoites of P. falciparum may infect all the red blood cell subpopulations, causing parasitemias of up to 50%, with high lethality.

The mechanisms of anemia are multifactoral and are not fully understood. The principles are as follows: hemolysis of parasitized red cells due to rupture of the schizonts; decline in the production of erythrocytes due to depression of erythropoiesis; increased phagocytosis of the red cells due to the change in sodium metabolism; and hemolysis of the parasitized or unparasitized red cells through immunologic mechanisms (16).

Disseminated intravascular coagulation is difficult to understand in malarial infection. Intravascular hemolysis of infected cells with release of thromboplastic materials, the exclusion of parasitized red cells, changes in permeability, and slowed blood flow in the capillaries may all lead to disseminated intravascular coagulation (DIC) (13, 17). The appearance of DIC coincides with a high degree of parasitemia, noticeable anemia, and pulmonary decompensation. The first signs are the appearance of petechiae, mainly in the conjunctiva, hemorrhagic suffusions in the skin, and, sometimes, hemorrhage (epistaxis or gastrointestinal hemorrhage).

Relapsing malaria caused by P. vivax (benign tertian malaria)

Malaria caused by P. vivax is characterized by its long-term development, intermittent fever with paroxysms on alternate days, anemia, and splenomegaly. Relapses may occur after a variable period of latency.

The incubation period generally varies from 10 to 18 days, but it may last from 8 to 11 months.

The primary attack begins with headache, fever, pain (mainly in the back), prostration, and nausea. In relapses or in patients who have already had malaria, such symptoms are mild or absent.

In individuals infected for the first time, the fever is irregular or remittent and lasts from two to four days. Subsequently it takes on the nature of a tertian fever, becoming intermittent on alternate days (Figure 4.8). The initial irregularity is due to the asynchronicity of parasites developing in the red cells and, consequently, the simultaneous presence in the blood of several populations of the parasite (2).

The paroxysms are complete, with well-defined periods of cold, heat, and sweating. They occur mainly in the afternoon, but they also may take place in the morning. Body temperature often rises above 40°C.

In general, the spleen is palpable and enlarged in patients who have had repeated infections. Hepatomegaly is also frequent.

Relapses are frequent after the initial attack. Although they may occur within an extremely variable period, they generally do so from 8 to 40 weeks after the first episode.

Although malaria caused by *P. vivax* in man may affect different organs and although there are always changes in the liver, it rarely develops into more serious forms. The most important complication, mainly in endemic regions, is secondary hypochromic anemia, which keeps the individual feeling weak up to a month after the infection is cured. Occasionally, there is also rupture of the spleen.

Soviet publications cite cases of fulminant malaria caused by *P. vivax*. It affects mainly children and young patients infected for the first time, and is characterized by the rapid development of symptoms and a high lethality. The patients exhibit a quick rise in temperature, severe headache, vomiting, convulsions, and death *(2)*.

Relapsing malaria caused by *P. ovale* (benign tertian ovale malaria)

This is characterized by intermittent fever, moderate splenomegaly, anemia, and a benign course. Patients frequently recover spontaneously after a few paroxysms.

The incubation period lasts from 11 to 16 days. Clinical signs of *P. ovale* malaria are similar to those of *P. vivax* malaria, although less severe. Less frequently than in malaria caused by *P. vivax*, the clinical signs begin with an irregular or remittent fever.

Paroxysms occur every 48 hours, generally after 6:00 p.m., and are not as frequent as those of *P. vivax* malaria (Figure 4.9). Chills are less intense, the body temperature never rises above 39.5°C, and the spleen does not become as enlarged.

The special characteristic of malaria caused by *P. ovale* is the high rate of spontaneous interruption of the paroxysms after the initial attack. Although it is rarely associated with complications, a moderate secondary anemia can often be detected.

Nonrelapsing malaria caused by *P. malariae* (quartan malaria)

This is characterized by an intermittent, frequently quartan, fever; mild anemia; splenomegaly; low parasitemia; and a lengthy development (Figure 4.10). Although there are no relapses, clinical recrudescences may occur after long periods of latency.

The incubation period of the naturally contracted infection varies from 18 to 40 days. The prodromic symptoms, which involve headache, general malaise, chills, and myalgias, are generally less severe than those of malaria caused by *P. vivax*.

A primary attack's clinical signs are similar to those of *P. vivax* malaria, with regular paroxysms every 72 hours. These usually occur in the afternoon, and the chill stage is not very intense. The anemia, if any, is mild; splenomegaly may be noticeable, with a palpable spleen, two weeks after the onset of clinical symptoms. The disease develops slowly and gradually.

Although recrudescences are most common during the first year, they may occur after much longer intervals (up to 52 years). The mechanisms governing these prolonged recrudescences are unknown, but the exoerythrocytic cycle is probably not involved. It is assumed that erythrocytic forms could survive in the host protected from the humeral and/or cellular immune response by means of a continuous antigenic variation *(1)*.

The nephrotic syndrome is the most important and frequent complication of this type of malaria in endemic areas. It probably develops from a lesion of the renal glomerulus caused by the deposit of immune complexes. The syndrome is characterized by a slow but progressive development, with high proteinuria and hypoproteinemia, noticeable edemas, arterial hypertension, and renal insufficiency.

MALARIA AND PREGNANCY

Complications of malaria develop twice as often in pregnant patients (2). During the first half of pregnancy the abortion rate is as high as 30%, and during the second half there is evidence of maternal immunosuppression, which tends to produce more serious, and commonly fatal, development. Factors leading to such immunosuppression include high levels of suprarenal steroids, chorionic gonadotropin, and alpha-fetoprotein (1, 18).

A pregnant woman may have a higher level of parasitemia (10 times greater than a nonpregnant patient). This is probably due to an inadequate immune response, mainly in patients infected for the first time, and it promotes complications in the infection's development.

From a clinical standpoint, malaria is similar in pregnant and nonpregnant patients. However, among the former, fever tends to be higher and the paroxysms may take longer to stabilize. In malaria caused by *P. falciparum* fever is continuous and tends to follow a more serious course, particularly among patients infected for the first time. Malaria causes susceptibility to toxemia of pregnancy, with preeclampsia and eclampsia. In pregnant patients, anemia associated with the infection causes abortion, premature birth, and low birth weight.

The mechanism causing congenital malaria is not understood. It is suggested that in nonimmune infected pregnant women there might be a lesion in the placenta that allows passage of the protozoan. Another possibility is contamination of the fetal blood at the time of birth, in which case the infection should be considered induced malaria.

The clinical characteristics of congenital malaria are similar to those of other perinatal infections. The newborn frequently may exhibit moderate fever, irritability, and anorexia. Although hepatosplenomegaly is observed, icterus is infrequent (19).

MALARIA IN CHILDREN

In children older than five years, malaria develops as in adults. However, preschool-age children do not manifest physical clinical signs characteristic of malarial paroxysm. This frequently leads to a mistaken diagnosis (2). In preschool-age children in endemic regions, malaria caused by *P. falciparum* is responsible for high mortality and morbidity rates (2, 6).

Children in hyperendemic areas do not normally contract malaria during the first two months of life because they have immunity transferred by the mother. Nevertheless, after the first year, most children can contract malaria. If the species responsible is *P. falciparum,* the infection's development may be serious.

Nursing babies generally do not exhibit typical paroxysms. They are flaccid and drowsy, they lose their appetite, and they are cold and may have vomiting and convulsions. Their body temperature varies from 38.5°C to 40°C, and fever may be continuous, remittent, intermittent, or irregular. Later there may be abdominal pain and diarrhea. The spleen and liver may be enlarged, but this is not frequent. If the development is more serious, icterus and anemia occur (2).

When malnutrition and other infections accompany malaria, as they commonly do, malaria's development may be more serious even when it is suitably treated.

In the disease's serious forms, the etiologic agent is generally *P. falciparum*. Coma is associated with paleness, convulsions, and vomiting. Occasionally there is abdominal pain and icterus. *P. vivax* malaria may become serious in children on rare occasions. In such instances, it begins with intense headache, nausea, vomiting, and convulsions and may be fatal (2).

In children who live in endemic areas and suffer from *P. malariae* malaria, a nephrotic syndrome, whose prognosis tends to be unfavorable, may develop.

INDUCED MALARIA

Malaria may be transmitted by inoculation of fresh blood from contaminated needles used by drug addicts or health services personnel. It may also be induced through transfusion of contaminated blood or blood products.

Any of the four kinds of human malaria may be induced through transfusions. The incubation period may be from 10 hours to 60 days and depends on the plasmodium species and the number of parasites injected. *P. falciparum* has the shortest incubation periods and *P. malariae* the longest (3).

The symptoms vary, with remittent fever, nausea, vomiting, myalgia, icterus, diarrhea, and abdominal pain. Malaria's typical paroxysms rarely occur. The disease is difficult to diagnose in immunosuppressed patients, and serious changes in the brain may develop (3).

TROPICAL SPLENOMEGALY SYNDROME

This syndrome occurs in malaria-endemic regions and is characterized by a pronounced splenomegaly, the absence of parasites in the peripheral blood, high serum IgM levels, increased levels of malaria antibodies, and a good response to prolonged antimalarial chemoprophylaxis.

As a pathogenic mechanism, it has been suggested that a defect in the suppressor cells could activate polyclonal B lymphocytes which, in turn, could also be induced by a mitogen associated with the parasite (16). This syndrome's high incidence in certain groups and families also suggests that its presence is influenced by genetic factors.

REFERENCES

(1) Bruce-Chwatt, L. J. *Essential Malariology*. London: W. Heinemann Medical Books, 1985.
(2) Loban, K. M., and E. S. Polozok. *Malaria*. Moscow: Mir Publishers, 1985.
(3) Bruce-Chwatt, L. J. Transfusion malaria revisited. *Trop Dis Bull* 79:827–840, 1982.
(4) Bruce-Chwatt, L. J. (ed.), R. H. Black, C. J. Canfield, D. F. Clyde, W. Peters, and W. H. Wernsdorfer. *Chemotherapy of Malaria*, 2nd edition. Monograph Series, No. 27. Geneva: World Health Organization, 1981.
(5) Hall, A. P. The treatment of severe falciparum malaria. *Trans R Soc Trop Med Hyg* 71:367–379, 1977.

(6) World Health Organization Malaria Action Program. Severe and complicated malaria. *Trans R Soc Trop Med Hyg* 80 (Suppl.), 1986.

(7) Schmutzhard, E., and F. Gerstenbrand. Cerebral malaria in Tanzania. Its epidemiology, clinical symptoms and neurological long-term sequelae in the light of 66 cases. *Trans R Soc Trop Med Hyg* 78:351–353, 1984.

(8) Looareesuwan, S., D. A. Warrell, N. J. White, P. Suntharasamai, M. J. Warrell, S. Chantaratherakitti, S. Changswek, L. Chongmankoncheep, and C. Kanchanaranya. Retinal haemorrhage, a common physical sign of prognostic significance in cerebral malaria. *Am J Trop Med Hyg* 32:911–915, 1983.

(9) Brooks, M. H., F. W. Kiel, T. W. Sheehy, and K. G. Barry. Acute pulmonary edema in falciparum malaria. A clinicopathological correlation. *N Eng J Med* 279:732–737, 1968.

(10) Applebaum, I. L., and M. Shrager. Pneumonitis associated with malaria. *Arch Int Med* 74:155–162, 1944.

(11) Maegraith, B. G. The liver in malaria and black-water fever. *In: Pathological Processes in Malaria and Black-water Fever*. Oxford: Blackwell Scientific Publications, 1948.

(12) Glenn, P. M., L. I. Kaplan, H. S. Read, and F. T. Becker. Clinical and laboratory studies of liver function in therapeutic malaria. *Am J Med Sci* 212:197–206, 1946.

(13) Boulos, M. Hepatic involvement in malaria: A clinical-biochemical-histopathological correlation. Thesis, School of Medicine, University of São Paulo, 1983.

(14) Ramachandran, S., and M. V. F. Perera. Jaundice and hepatomegaly in primary malaria. *J Trop Med Hyg* 79:207–210, 1976.

(15) Weatherall, D. J., and S. Abdalla. The anaemia of *Plasmodium falciparum* malaria. *Br Med Bull* 38:147–151, 1982.

(16) Perrin, L. H., L. J. Mackey, and P. A. Miescher. The hematology of malaria in man. *Semin Hematol* 19:70–82, 1982.

(17) Hernández, A. D., and P. H. Rodríguez. La coagulación intravascular diseminada como complicación del paludismo falciparum. *Rev Cubana Med Trop* 34:239–247, 1982.

(18) Covell, G. Congenital malaria. *Trop Dis Bull* 47:1147–1167, 1950.

(19) Thompson, D., C. Pegelow, A. Underman, and D. Powars. Congenital malaria: a rare cause of splenomegaly and anemia in an American infant. *Pediatrics* 60:209–212, 1977.

Chapter 5

MICROSCOPIC DIAGNOSIS OF MALARIAL PARASITES IN THE BLOOD[1]

Francisco J. López-Antuñano

Blood is the medium in which the malarial parasites are found. Since it is the vehicle that brings the *Plasmodium* into the microscopic field, the person who will be looking for parasites should know something about it.

The blood basically consists of a liquid called plasma in which the cellular components—erythrocytes, platelets, and leukocytes—are suspended. These elements develop in the bone marrow and are released into the peripheral circulation as the organism requires. The cellular part of the blood includes a variety of components that not only provide the laboratory technician with information about the patient but also are of help in judging the quality of the preparation and staining.[2] Both the blood and the parasites in it are damaged by desiccation.

When whole blood is allowed to stand in a test tube it coagulates. Unless it is spread quickly, a drop of blood on a slide will coagulate in the same way. This affects the manner in which the preparation adheres to the slide. If the blood is stirred after coagulation begins, areas of different thicknesses and concentrations will be produced, and these can be easily recognized by examination with the microscope's low-power objective. The leukocytes will be seen in strings or clumps instead of the regular, uniform distribution they present in a promptly spread preparation.

THE CELLULAR ELEMENTS

The erythrocytes, or red blood cells, are biconcave disks that appear singly, grouped at random, or in rolls like stacks of coins, called "rouleaux." They are dark yellow because of their hemoglobin content. When fresh unstained blood is pressed under a coverslip, the erythrocytes can be compressed or highly distorted without being damaged structurally. Against this background the parasites, if they are present, can be recognized only if they are old enough to contain pigment. Therefore, the examination of fresh blood is not practical.

The erythrocytes are derived from bone marrow cells, and they contain a nucleus in their early stages. Shortly before the developing erythrocytes are released into the circulation, the nucleus is lost and the young red cells of various sizes may contain blue-staining components clearly visible in well-stained smears. Different authors

---

[1]Revised version of parts I.3 through I.5 of the *Manual for the Microscopic Diagnosis of Malaria*, 4th edition (Scientific Publication No. 276), Washington, D.C., Pan American Health Organization, 1975.

[2]All staining of blood samples mentioned in the chapter was done with derivatives of Romanowsky's method.

have described them variously as *reticulum* (from reticulocytes), *polychromasia*, or *punctate basophilia*. These elements all disappear one to three days after the red cells enter the bloodstream. After dehemoglobinization (release of hemoglobin through the action of aqueous solutions) and staining of thick blood films, bluish masses can be observed in the otherwise clear spaces between the leukocytes. These masses range from the size of a small lymphocyte to that of a large polymorphonuclear leukocyte. They consist of reticulocytes and are called cell remains. Their appearance varies from a fine haze or mottled cloudiness to a group of dense blue dots of variable size. Normal blood contains from one to three per microscopic field, but they may be countless when malaria or another infection has caused severe anemia, forcing the bone marrow to produce enormous quantities of immature cells.

The appearance of fresh red blood cells may change greatly in accordance with the changing conditions of their surroundings. In serum or in a 0.85% sodium chloride solution, their smooth circular shape is maintained. If the amount of salt is increased to 1.5%, a cell will develop small protuberances all over its outer surface, making it look like a submarine contact mine. These crenated cells may retain this appearance even after staining. An excess or shortage of salt in the solution causes red cells to rupture and release their hemoglobin, whereby the water in the solution turns reddish.

Platelets have no nucleus, since they originate from the cytoplasm of a very large bone marrow cell called a megakaryocyte. On the same slide they may appear as separate elements or in groups of different densities. The color may range from pink to violet (never blue) in different samples. They vary so much in size and shape that in blood that has dried slowly or been defibrinated they take almost any form. If the slides remained unstained for a long time, the platelets may stain so intensely that they hide small parasites.

When unstained, the leukocytes or white blood cells are transparent and highly refractile, and their cytoplasm may show movement. After staining, the nucleus becomes bluish violet. They vary in size and shape, and their cytoplasm may contain granules, in which case they are called granulocytes, or may not, giving them the name agranulocytes. The polymorphonuclear cells vary in appearance from compact, well defined, and well stained to large, pale, irregular, and distorted.

There are two kinds of agranulocytes: lymphocytes and monocytes. The lymphocytes contain a single mass of nuclear material which is rounded and usually well defined. The cytoplasm stains a pale blue color, is somewhat transparent, and may contain a few bright red granules. The small lymphocytes, which measure 8 to 10 micrometers in diameter, are the most uniform cells in the blood. They are very important to the microscopist because they serve as a basis for comparison to determine the size of parasites in a thick blood film, just as the red blood cells do in thin smears (Figure 5.1). Like lymphocytes, the monocytes also have a single mass of nuclear material, and their cytoplasm, which is denser, stains blue. Their numbers increase at the beginning of a malaria infection. As active phagocytes, they can take in not only the malarial pigment but also the red blood cells that contain mature malaria parasites, including schizonts. Their cytoplasm shows a fine bluish gray stroma, and their nuclei have a more or less prominent cleft.

The granulocytes, or polymorphonuclear leukocytes, are so called due to their lobed nuclei and the granules in their cytoplasm. There are three kinds, recognized by the way their granules stain. The neutrophils' granules may be blue, pink, or violet and are irregular in size, shape, and distribution. With poor staining, the cytoplasm may turn so red that an inexperienced microscopist may erroneously classify them as eosinophils. The latter, by contrast, have granules that are so large and so regular in size, shape, and compactness that they can even be identified before staining, when the nuclei cannot be distinguished. The compact granules themselves should stain a dark copperish red rather than the familiar bright red characteristic of eosin-stained tissue sections. If it were necessary to choose a single feature by which to judge staining quality, it might well be the appearance of these granules. In the case of the third kind of granulocyte, the basophils, the granules are coarse, regular in size, and usually stain deep blue. Since they are rarely seen in normal blood, they are of no assistance to the microscopist in diagnosing malaria or in evaluating the staining.

Figure 5.1 shows some of the blood elements that are normally observed in a thick film.

GENERAL CHARACTERISTICS OF THE PLASMODIUM SPECIES THAT INFECT HUMAN BLOOD

Like any other animal species, plasmodia vary in size, shape, and appearance according to their development stage and individual characteristics. In general, the plasmodia of the four species that normally parasitize human red blood cells are very similar and could be mistaken for one another, with the exception of the gametocytes of *Plasmodium falciparum*, which generally assume the crescent "banana" or "sausage" shape. Nevertheless, when a thick blood film is allowed to dry slowly, the gametocytes of *P. falciparum* often become rounded and on occasion exflagellate, in which case they may be confused with gametocytes of the other species.

To accurately identify species of *Plasmodium* by microscopic blood examination, it is necessary to observe a sufficient number of different forms to get an idea of the pattern of variation constant for each species. It is not enough to memorize a list of colors, shapes, and certain morphological features that have been attributed to various species of the parasite and to parasitized red cells. These descriptions are not always valid because they do not reflect the natural shape of the parasite inside the erythrocyte, but rather are artifacts of the blood sample preparation, especially in thin blood smears, in which the parasitized erythrocytes are pressed and the parasites' original shape changed. This is the origin of the so-called "band" forms seen in a smear of blood parasitized by *P. malariae*, which never appear in a thick film prepared with the same blood taken at the same time from the same patient.

Whoever examines the samples must be observant and take note of the variety of parasitic forms that can be seen in each of the plasmodium species that infect humans. This person must be trained not only to recognize the variations in form of the different species of parasites but also the variations caused by differing conditions under which the blood sample was obtained.

Each time a parasitic form comes into focus, the examiner must ask himself three questions:

    1. Is this a plasmodium?

    2. How many plasmodia are there in this blood sample?

3. Do the forms fall within the pattern of variation that can be expected for the species in question?

The answer to the first question can be obtained by examining enough microscopic fields to find a parasite that can be viewed in full detail and unequivocably identified. The color and density of the nucleus' chromatin, the appearance of the cytoplasm, and whether it contains malarial pigment, or hemozoin, are then assessed. If the form to be identified does not resemble the unmistakably identified parasite in these attributes, it probably is not a genuine plasmodium. The question is simplified if the organism's image is mentally located in its appropriate place within the development cycle.

Figures 5.2 and 5.3 depict schematically part of the erythrocytic cycle as observed in the peripheral blood for the three most common species of plasmodia that infect humans.

It should always be borne in mind that examination of a blood sample for plasmodia is not very sensitive if only a few parasites are present (less than 10 per microliter of blood). A thick blood film of 1.0 to 1.5 cm^2 area could contain from 500 to 800 satisfactory microscopic fields (total magnification of 700–800 diameters with an oil immersion objective).

An entire blood preparation is examined only under very special circumstances, such as in studies of experimental infections or to evaluate the effect of drugs on the plasmodia. When a febrile patient's symptoms are due to malaria, parasites can be found in abundance, with possibly one or more in each microscopic field.

Routinely, at least 100 microscopic fields are examined in a uniform, well-dehemoglobinized, and well-stained thick blood film. If the preparation varies in thickness, dehemoglobinization, or staining, the number of fields examined must be increased in keeping with the sample's quality.

It is usually important and necessary to estimate the number of parasites present. In the first place, from a practical standpoint, a species is most likely to be identified correctly on the basis of a large number of parasites. Secondly, a microscopic diagnosis can be reviewed more precisely when the parasite densities are noted. Finally, the systematic recording of parasite densities helps epidemiologists calculate the proportion of high parasitemias and therefore be aware of a recent transmission.

The estimated parasite density per microliter of blood can be based on the number of parasites per 100 microscopic fields or the number of parasites per 100 leukocytes. In the former instance, it must be taken into account that 100 microscopic fields of a well-prepared thick blood film examined at 750 × magnification corresponds to approximately 0.2 microliters of blood. Thus, one parasite per microscopic field means an average of 100 parasites per 100 fields, or 500 parasites per microliter.

The second method consists of finding the number of parasites per 100 leukocytes in a stained thick blood film. Under certain circumstances, this count can be obtained at the same time a leukocyte count is done with a Newbauer hemocytometer. Once the number of parasites per 100 leukocytes and the number of leukocytes per microliter are known, it is easy to determine the number of parasites per microliter. If the actual leukocyte count is not available, as is often the case with samples from the field, an average number of leukocytes per microliter may be used (preferably an age-group average). Parasitemias of more than 1,000 per microliter are considered high, and those of less than 1,000 are considered low.

BROODS

In malarial infections, broods are the unsynchronized parasite population bursts found in the peripheral blood.

The four species associated with human malaria require some minimum period to complete schizogony. This is true in both the hepatic and erythrocytic cycles, and the periods vary depending on the species. Schizogony may be delayed by a few days in the liver, and may be delayed or advanced a few hours in the peripheral blood. As a consequence of these variations, parasites at different stages of development may be found in the blood. However, not all the different stages are necessarily seen in routine thick film examinations, since there are sometimes too few to be found in the microscopic fields examined.

Whenever a sufficient number of parasites complete schizogony and enter the peripheral blood of a nonimmune or semi-immune patient at the same time, or within a few hours of each other, clinical symptoms are produced. When one brood predominates, the symptoms appear every 48 hours in infections caused by P. falciparum, P. vivax, and P. ovale and every 72 hours in infections caused by P. malariae. The paroxysms indicate that the parasites are completing schizogony within a few hours of each other in sufficient numbers to cause symptoms of the disease. When the paroxysms occur daily, they indicate the presence of two or more broods. In fact, at the beginning of an attack a patient may experience daily paroxysms, meaning that the classic signs and symptoms of infection are "out of sync" owing to the superimposition of another pattern by at least one additional brood. Nevertheless, this situation does not usually persist because once the dominant brood is established, the parasites of the other brood(s) are suppressed and consequently cease being abundant enough to cause symptoms.

Broods may arise from: 1) the release of hepatic merozoites in the bloodstream at different times; 2) the release of erythrocytic merozoites at different times owing to advanced or delayed development of the parasites inside the red cells; or 3) a new sporozoite infection caused by the bite of an infected mosquito before immunity is established (Figure 5.4).

CHARACTERISTICS OF THE INDIVIDUAL SPECIES OF PLASMODIUM THAT INFECT HUMAN BLOOD

There are differences in the behavior of the individual species that are reflected not only in the symptoms they cause in the patient but also in the forms seen in the blood.

PLASMODIUM FALCIPARUM

Apparently, the mere presence of the merozoite inside the red cell changes its external layer or membrane. It is known that this phenomenon is not due to any specific property of the cell, since the merozoites of P. falciparum penetrate young and old red blood cells indiscriminately, whereas P. vivax shows a preference for young cells and P. malariae for old cells.

Parasites in tissue sections will not show the characteristic features seen in parasitized cells in a well-stained blood sample. The actual parasites, with their customary hematoxylin and eosin staining, are rarely seen, but their presence is indicated by the amount of malarial pigment proportional to the parasite's size during life. Chromatin and cytoplasm can often be distinguished in material that has been placed promptly in the appropriate fixative and then stained. The results of the staining depend on how soon after death the tissue samples are taken, or how quickly the cadaver has been refrigerated. The best results have been obtained from Tomlinson's technique *(1)*.

Examination of any tissue, especially cerebral tissue, will show how the parasitized red cells attach themselves to the walls of the small blood vessels wherever blood flow and pressure are low. In the smaller vessels, where there is little or no turbulence, these parasitized red blood cells are not dislodged. Thus, the walls of a small venule may be completely covered with parasitized red cells while at the same time few if any parasites are seen among the numerous red cells in the vessel's lumen (Figures 5.5A and B).

At autopsy, it can be seen that each of the red blood cells adhering to the capillary lining has a granule of pigment representing the residue of what was a living parasite. Further evidence that the parasitized cells attach themselves to the endothelial lining is that none of the red cells involved in petechial hemorrhages from a ruptured capillary contain parasites (Figure 5.5C). With the red cells' well-known ability to accommodate themselves to a variety of constrictions and obstructions, those that are not parasitized can move around the fixed cells inside the capillary as long as some pressure exists (Figure 5.5D). If the damage to the lining cells is too serious, the healthy red cells escape through the resultant opening. When the endothelium remains intact, no hemorrhages occur.

The foregoing explanation easily accounts for why only the asexual ring forms of the parasite are found in the peripheral blood. Only when shock develops can embolic phenomena be observed, apparently due to a lack of muscle tone in the vascular walls that enables the lightly adhered cells to move from the lining and clump together.

The high level of parasitemia characteristic of infections caused by *P. falciparum* can be explained by the fact that these blood vessels, whose lining is occupied by parasitized cells, are also full of uninfected cells. From their position inside fixed red cells, schizonts release merozoites, which are literally pressed against hundreds of cells. One or more merozoites quickly enter the closest red cell, regardless of whether it is young, old, or middle-aged.

Figures 5.6 to 5.11 show the great variety in number and size of the ring forms observed in peripheral blood during infections caused by *P. falciparum*. Even when two or more broods of asexual parasites are present, the only forms observed are ring forms and occasionally mature schizonts in severe cases.

It is thought that the gametocytes of *P. falciparum* grow and develop inside red blood cells that bind themselves in a similar way to the endothelium. However, upon maturation the gametocytes become elongated and the erythrocyte containing them breaks free and enters the circulation.

In a primary attack of *P. falciparum* malaria, parasitemia can be observed in the blood around the tenth or twelfth day, and symptoms appear within the following

24 hours. If the host is ready for the development of gametocytes, they will begin to appear 8 or 10 days later. If the case continues untreated, ring forms and gametocytes may persist together for several days or weeks, until the acquired immunity is sufficient to eliminate the asexual forms. After the asexual forms have been eliminated, no more gametocytes are produced, although those already present may continue circulating for five to seven more weeks.

Figure 5.12 shows four different behavior patterns of gametocytes in infections caused by *P. falciparum*. Since the cases represented were infections induced for the purpose of experimental chemotherapy studies, the precise dates of inoculation, beginning and end of the prepatent period, and the onset and clearance of the patent asexual and sexual parasitemia are known, as are dates of intermediate variations. Chloroquine, quinine, and pyrimethamine-sulfadoxine were used in these experiments as schizonticides, and primaquine was used as a gametocide.

On the basis of these studies, it can be concluded that the gametocytes represented in Figure 5.12:

- Generally appear during the second week of the patent asexual parasitemia.
- Disappear spontaneously five to seven weeks after clearance of the asexual forms.
- Remain in the bloodstream the entire time the patient suffers recrudescences of asexual parasitemia.
- Disappear within 72 hours after the administration of primaquine-type drugs, even in the presence of asexual forms.
- Do not appear at all when schizontocidal drugs are administered alone as soon as the asexual forms become patent.

Therefore, it is necessary for infections caused by *P. falciparum* to be treated radically with both schizonticides and gametocides to eliminate the infection and stop transmission.

P. falciparum infections normally show three phases: 1) only asexual (ring) forms (Figures 5.6 to 5.11); 2) asexual (ring) and sexual (gametocyte) forms together (a mixture of Figures 5.6 to 5.11, 5.13, and 5.14); or 3) only gametocytes (Figures 5.13 and 5.14). The latter two figures illustrate the appearance of small and large quantities of the gametocytes of *P. falciparum*.

An individual who is learning to identify the various species should have access to at least a dozen different blood samples showing the three phases. Each parasite should be studied carefully until as many ring forms of *P. falciparum* as possible have been observed. An effort should be made to learn the maximum degree of variation in number, size, and stage of development of the parasites that can occur in peripheral blood. It is important to keep the latter factor in mind in case more developed forms are seen, which would mean that the infection is more likely due to *P. vivax* or *P. malariae*.

The ring forms of *P. falciparum* can be small (Figures 5.6 and 5.7), medium (Figures 5.8 and 5.9), or large (Figures 5.10 and 5.11). A high proportion of small ring forms indicates the approach of schizogony. If the proportion of large forms is higher, the overall number of parasites will decline noticeably within six hours. It is important to understand that when an infection involves a single brood, the parasites may not be patent during intervals of several hours. However, single-brood infections are rare in semi-immune persons. When more than one brood of *P. falciparum* is present at the same time, the parasites are never absent from the peripheral blood, but their numbers may vary considerably.

PLASMODIUM VIVAX

The word "*vivax*" means lively, and it accurately describes the almost frenetic activity this species frequently exhibits. The *P. vivax* merozoite clearly prefers younger red blood cells, which are more elastic than mature ones and thus better able to enlarge so as to accommodate the growing parasite. Since red blood cells parasitized by *P. vivax* do not adhere to the vessel lining as do those parasitized by *P. falciparum*, the parasitized cells circulate freely at all times during the erythrocytic cycle or series of such cycles as schizogony takes place. The time the released *P. vivax* merozoites require to find a new host cell is much longer than that observed for *P. falciparum*. Moreover, the number of *P. vivax* parasites lost to phagocytosis is much greater. Consequently, parasitemias never reach the intensities achieved by *P. falciparum*. In their haste to find new shelter, the *P. vivax* merozoites may sometimes invade a cell already occupied by one, two, or more of their species. It is not unusual to find two chromatin fragments in young parasites, one of them frequently much smaller than the other.

The young *P. vivax* parasite moves around freely inside the red blood cell, putting out cytoplasmic pseudopodia to all areas of the cell. This gives rise to the appearance of strange forms so numerous and varied that only a few of them can be illustrated (Figures 5.15 to 5.22). It is possible that the large irregular parasite may not be recognized in its entirety in a thick blood film, since several compact portions of cytoplasm are frequently present. Although all of these may contain pigment, only one, perhaps the largest, has chromatin. The other portions may be overlooked because the small bridges of cytoplasm connecting them to the chromatin-containing part are too thin to be seen. The confusion that so often occurs in identifying *P. vivax* and *P. malariae* stems from the fact that the dense portion containing the chromatin is mistaken for a complete parasite. In order to appreciate what a complete parasite looks like in a thick film, it is often necessary to consider everything inside a diameter as large or larger than a small lymphocyte (6 to 8 μm) seen in the same blood (Figure 5.23).

In the case of *P. vivax*, the red cell membrane, rather than becoming sticky, produces a series of granules in its stroma. These granules, known as Schüffner's dots, are uniform in size, shape, and distribution. Fine at first, they become larger and more prominent until they sometimes seem to fill the cell, surrounding the maturing schizont. After staining they become reddish. In the thick film, especially at the periphery, this staining phenomenon sometimes appears as a pinkish halo around the parasites that is about the same size and shape as the host cell. This is called Schüffner's staining. Unless one of the modifications of Romanowsky's method is used in staining, well-defined dots can rarely be distinguished. Schüffner's dots occur only in infections caused by *P. vivax* and *P. ovale*. Their presence and not their absence should be used for identification purposes, since demonstration of this phenomenon requires a certain level of quality in staining and only some routinely stained slides show these changes.

A pinkish halo or shadow is also sometimes seen around the *P. falciparum* parasites and should not be confused with Schüffner's dots. When it appears in thick films, it is generally because they have been overstained or because the stain intensity varies or has faded. Species diagnosis should always be based on the total variety of developmental forms observed in infected blood and not on the appearance of individual stained components.

No phenomenon of this nature has been observed with *P. malariae* parasites in thick films.

As it matures, the *P. vivax* parasite becomes rounder and more regular, and its adult mononuclear asexual form, or preschizont, so resembles the gametocyte that it is not easy to tell them apart. The gametocytes appear when the asexual parasitemia is patent.

Unlike those of *P. falciparum*, the *P. vivax* gametocytes grow in the peripheral blood and are found in the circulation before they are completely developed. These developing sexual forms of *P. vivax* have compact, dense cytoplasm, ordinarily with considerable pigment, and are sometimes mistaken for *P. malariae*. Unlike those of *P. falciparum*, the gametocytes of *P. vivax* and *P. malariae* disappear from circulation along with the asexual forms when a schizonticide is administered. However, there is no reason to confuse *P. vivax* gametocytes with those of *P. malariae*, especially in view of the latter's scarcity.

Although all growth stages of *P. vivax* may be represented in a single drop of blood, parasites representing two-thirds of the complete development cycle are normally observed at any given time. A mature schizont contains 14 to 24 merozoites just before it bursts. If two or more broods coexist, all of the parasite's stages can be found in a single blood sample. Therefore, it is superfluous to identify the parasitic forms as trophozoites, schizonts, and gametocytes, since all these forms can be present. Although it is sometimes claimed that ring forms of *P. vivax* can be found alone, this is not true in practice. A careful examination will reveal numerous small irregular forms never found in *P. falciparum*, and will probably also show advanced mononuclear forms and even schizonts. Whether the ring, irregular, large mononuclear forms, or schizonts predominate will depend on the time the blood sample is taken and the number of developing broods.

So-called "mixed" infections rarely exist clinically and occur as such during the 24- to 48-hour period in which the two species present struggle for dominance. Normally, *P. falciparum* dominates *P. vivax* and *P. vivax* dominates *P. malariae*. It is unusual to find any combination other than *P. vivax* accompanied by *P. falciparum* gametocytes. If a mixed infection is detected, the observed number of parasites for each species should be indicated. The subordinate species is noted after the dominant one. For example " + + + F 9V" means that there are more than 20 *P. falciparum* rings per microscopic field and nine *P. vivax* parasites per 100 fields.[3]

PLASMODIUM MALARIAE

This species occurs in regions in which the preceding two species are found, but is less prevalent and as a rule is subordinate to them. Since its gametocytes are

---

[3] See Chapter 9, Laboratory Techniques.

normally scarce, their transmission is not as frequent as with the other species. The preerythrocytic period lasts 11 days, and the parasites can be seen in the blood at any time between 19 and 30 days. The persistence of *P. malariae* infections is well known. One reported case has been active for 52 years, but since modern schizonticides are very efficient, infections of such long duration are unlikely to occur in the future.

As with *P. vivax*, the infected cells circulate freely in the peripheral blood. However, in contrast to the other species, *P. malariae* merozoites prefer to infect the oldest red blood cells. This characteristic, together with an average schizogony of 8 to 12 divisions, results in a lower total parasitemia than in the case of *P. vivax*. The 50% increase in time necessary for it to achieve complete development and its distinctly slower activity compared with *P. vivax* bring about an earlier and more intense concentration of pigment.

Once inside the cell, the *P. malariae* parasite remains relatively immobile and does not extrude pseudopodia. On occasion, advanced presegmentation forms show some irregularity owing to the donut shape of the red blood cell that encloses the parasite. The entire parasite may be lodged in the peripheral tubular part of the biconcave disks of red blood cells that contain less than a normal amount of hemoglobin. Similar forms are found in infections caused by *P. vivax* that have persisted long enough to reduce hematocrit and hemoglobin values. If a single brood predominates in a *P. malariae* infection, a smaller proportion of the complete erythrocytic cycle is observed than in infections caused by *P. vivax* (Figures 5.24 to 5.27). When all the cycle's phases are found in a single blood specimen, it means that more than two broods of the parasite are present (Figure 5.4).

From the time just after the end of the ring stage until maturation of the schizonts, the *P. malariae* parasite is characterized by its density, intense pigmentation, and uniform, compact, and regular shape. Although a type of granulation has been described, this phenomenon is not routinely observed even in excellent thick film preparations.

It is not uncommon for 1% to 4% of the parasites observed in an infection caused by *P. falciparum* or *P. vivax* to be classified as "undoubted" *P. malariae*. This can result when a blood sample containing only *P. falciparum* gametocytes dries very slowly, giving the parasites time to assume a round form. If such forms are numerous, they may be mistaken for *P. malariae*.

PLASMODIUM OVALE

Infections produced by this parasite rarely occur in the Americas. They are frequently observed in East Africa, the Middle East, Malaysia, Indonesia, and the Philippines, and are especially common in tropical Africa.

The exoerythrocytic stage lasts nine days, and precisely on the ninth day after infection the merozoites penetrate young red blood cells. Like *P. vivax* and *P. malariae*, the *P. ovale* parasites circulate freely and develop in the bloodstream, completing their erythrocytic cycle in 48 hours. The parasitemias are usually low. In stained thick blood films, the parasites look like a cross of two species: *P. malariae* parasites with the Schüffner's dots characteristic of *P. vivax* (also called James' dots in *P. ovale* infections). Although in *P. ovale* the dots may be less numerous than in *P. vivax*, they are more pronounced and tend to overshadow the parasite. Additional chromatin is as frequent as in *P. vivax*.

This species is characterized by the oval and fimbriated shape of red cells that contain parasites. However, this phenomenon is not easy to observe. Even on a thin smear it can only be seen when the humidity is high and the blood sample has been dried quickly. This species is therefore very difficult to identify in a thick film unless the observer has had the opportunity to work in countries where it is frequently seen. When anemia is present in prolonged *P. vivax* infections, the parasites inside red blood cells containing insufficient hemoglobin can take on a form that makes them difficult to distinguish from *P. ovale*. Therefore, it is risky for inexperienced personnel to attempt to identify the parasite only by its morphology. Only if the supposed *P. ovale* is transferred, either by inoculation or by a mosquito bite, to another person and if the resulting infection follows the *P. ovale* pattern may diagnosis of *P. ovale* infection be certified in areas in which this species does not normally exist. If by chance fimbriated red cells are observed in a suspected *P. vivax* infection in a blood sample taken close to schizogony, repeated samples may show behavior not corresponding to *P. vivax*.

Infections caused by *P. falciparum* and *P. vivax* dominate those caused by *P. ovale*. The latter, which originally were considered somewhat innocuous, have been shown to be as serious as infections caused by *P. vivax*. Parasitemias may persist for months.

REFERENCES

(1) Boyd, M. F. *Malariology*. Philadelphia and London: W. B. Saunders Company, 1949.
(2) Pan American Health Organization. *Manual for the Microscopic Diagnosis of Malaria*, 4th ed. Scientific Publication No. 276. Washington, D.C.: PAHO, 1973.

Chapter 6

DETECTION OF MALARIA PARASITES IN THE MOSQUITO BY MICROSCOPIC OBSERVATION

Janine M. Ramsey

An anopheline mosquito that feeds on blood containing malaria parasites will generally become infected (1). The adult female mosquito, the definitive host of the plasmodium, is the site where the sexual cycle of the parasite takes place. Gametocytes ingested by the mosquito during the blood meal undergo fertilization, followed by ookinete migration through the mosquito midgut, oocyst maturation, and, finally, release of sporozoites which migrate to the salivary glands. The mosquito may then transmit the parasite to man.

The major efforts of malaria eradication and control programs are directed against the adult insect. These interventions attempt to interrupt either infection of the mosquito or parasite transmission to the vertebrate host, in this case, man.

A primary reason to diagnose the presence of malaria parasites in a mosquito is to identify naturally occurring vectors (2, 3). To be a vector, it is not enough that a mosquito species be capable of acquiring infection, that the species be anthropophilic, or that it occur at a high density. Many species have been experimentally infected, but do not become infective (4, 5). Conversely, certain strains of mosquitoes may show little or no susceptibility to human parasites under experimental conditions, but circumstantial data from the field may implicate them as potential vectors (6). Although many mosquito species, including *Aedes* and *Culex*, are anthropophilic, only certain species within the genus *Anopheles* actually transmit human malaria (7, 8). In turn, many zoophilic anopheline species can be important vectors of human malaria (9). In order to adequately understand how transmission occurs in a given area, the species of mosquito that play a primary or secondary role in transmission must be defined. The differing importance of various subspecies within the *Anopheles gambiae* complex in different regions in Africa is an excellent example of this requirement, because, as pointed out by Coluzzi (10), determination of the vectorial capacity of each of these subspecies, as well as other potential vectors, has a direct impact on entomological control measures. The intervention program can focus on the identified vector or vectors, and its success can be monitored by evaluating infection or infectivity in the mosquito population.

Another reason for investigating the plasmodia infection rate in mosquito species is to define which local species are capable of infection and transmission of the parasite in the study area, even though they may not yet be known to be naturally infected. Control measures directed against a given species could result in a change in the relative importance of primary or secondary vectors, or even the emergence of new ones. Experimental infection studies can evaluate the infectivity potential of alternative species (11, 12).

A third reason to identify the presence of parasites in mosquitoes is to determine the susceptibility of these species to infection via a blood meal and the capacity of the species to transmit infection based on its physiology and genetics (13, 14). These experimental infections are also used to determine the parameters in the vertebrate host that influence the infectivity to the mosquito. These parameters could include gametocytemia, mature gametocyte ratios, effect of antibodies and complement (15–19), and parasite strain differences (20–24).

Methods utilized to detect or diagnose the presence of malaria parasites in mosquitoes either find and identify the whole parasite by direct microscopic observation or identify one or more specific protein components of the parasite by immunologic assay. This chapter describes the methodology used for observation of intact parasites.

MOSQUITO DISSECTION

The original and most widely used method to determine the presence of parasites in mosquitoes is dissection. Parasites can be found mainly in the post-zygotic stages, that is, as early-to-late oocysts on the mosquito midgut or as sporozoites that have been released from the oocysts and are either migrating in the hemolymph or already in the salivary glands. Many excellent manuals exist describing dissection methods for the midgut and salivary glands (8, 25–28). A diagram is included in Figure 6.1, but it should be noted that any method is only a guide and that each individual will eventually develop his or her particular technique.

The choice of which organ to dissect from the mosquito will depend on the type of data required. To determine whether a mosquito has become infected, the midgut is dissected to investigate the presence of oocysts, their number, stage of development, and positioning on the midgut (6, 29–32). If oocysts are observed, the mosquito is considered "infected." However, in order to determine whether a mosquito is "infective," the salivary glands must be dissected and examined for the presence of sporozoites (33). Number of sporozoites and the number of infected lobes of the salivary glands should be noted. Since it is quite common in natural infections for only one lobe to contain sporozoites, all lobes of the gland must be viewed in order to determine whether parasites are present in a given mosquito.

Once the mosquito has been dissected and the desired organs are exposed on a slide in saline or buffer solution, various methods can be used to find the parasite. The most common method used is that of observation with the light microscope. A cover slip is placed on the drop of saline or buffer solution containing the mosquito organs and the slide is placed on the microscope stage. Generally, oocysts on the midgut can be observed with a $10\times$ objective. An inexperienced observer may require a $40\times$ objective to view sporozoites. In both cases, the ocular should be 7 to $10\times$. If immediate observation is not required, the tissues can be allowed to dry, then fixed and stained with Giemsa or Romanowsky's stain for mounting and later study.

Once the parasites have been detected, several methods are available to study them further. Entire salivary glands, midguts, or the liberated sporozoites can be fixed and prepared for transmission or scanning electron microscopy (34). Since the sporozoites of one species are indistinguishable morphologically from those of another with a light microscope, liberated sporozoites can be dried onto slides and later analyzed using specific antibodies for each species in an immunofluorescence assay (35), enzyme-linked immunosorbent assay (36), or radioimmunoassay (37).

Data acquired from the dissection of mosquitoes that were collected in an endemic area may be analyzed for various epidemiological purposes. The identification of sporozoites in the salivary glands of any mosquito species implicates that species as a potential vector. Once it is known to be a vector, dissection can allow determination of the sporozoite rate or index, which is the percentage of the population of dissected mosquitoes whose salivary glands are found to contain sporozoites. The sporozoite index can be used in various mathematical models to determine the theoretical entomological inoculation rate, vectorial capacity, and the corresponding level of transmission (33, 38–40).[1]

The advantage of using dissection, as opposed to other methods, to diagnose the presence of parasites is that individual salivary glands can be examined to find out the proportion of infective mosquitoes. The disadvantages of the method are that it is time consuming, requires a certain level of technical skill, and is an inefficient approach when infection rates are low. For those reasons, data on sporozoite indices from endemic areas are almost completely lacking.

MOSQUITO FILTRATION

Alternate methods that allow the processing of larger numbers of mosquitoes have been developed in recent years. The filtration method requires maceration of the whole body or the thorax of mosquitoes in batches of up to 100, depending on the number of specimens collected. The sporozoites are isolated from mosquito tissues and observed by microscopy (39). Although this method allows determination of the infection rate, it does not establish the exact proportion of the sample that was actually infective.

The method[2] consists of passing the macerated mosquito tissues through a glass wool plug and then through a Whatman #2 paper filter. The filtrate is then fixed with glutaraldehyde and centrifuged to concentrate the tissues in a small volume. The resuspended precipitate is passed through another Whatman #2 filter. The sample is then ready for observation with phase microscopy.

This method is useful in epidemiological surveys (41) since it permits large numbers of mosquitoes to be processed rapidly and an overall infection rate to be calculated. This rate can then be used to determine how many mosquitoes would have to be dissected to find at least one positive. Subsequent dissection of an appropriate number of mosquitoes could provide the sporozoite index. Although the infection rate is not useful in current transmission models, it can be used to monitor mosquito populations in an area where control measures are under way.

The filtration method is technically simple except for final observation with the microscope, which requires a trained eye that can distinguish sporozoites from fragments of mosquito tissue resulting from the maceration process. Unfortunately, like the dissection method, it does not allow the species of parasite to be identified.

---

[1] For practical application of these mathematical models, the study sample must be representative of the different mosquito populations that are involved in transmission.
[2] See Chapter 9, Laboratory Techniques.

OTHER METHODS FOR ISOLATING PARASITES IN THE VECTOR

Multiple methods have been developed to study parasitological and biochemical aspects of the infective stage of plasmodia. Procedures have been designed to isolate, purify, and concentrate the sporozoites from large numbers of mosquitoes (42–47). These methods, which enable easy, large-scale isolation of sporozoites for use in immunization experiments or biochemical analysis, utilize the parasite's physical properties in sucrose and diatrizoate sodium gradients for separation from mosquito tissues. In addition, passage of infected mosquito macerates through filters or on DEAE-cellulose columns has been used to isolate masses of purified sporozoites.

Other experimental studies of the parasite in the vector have sought to measure the infective capacity of sporozoites other than those contained in the salivary glands (48). Although the mosquito can only transmit the parasite by injecting it from the salivary glands through the proboscis, mature sporozoites, even in the oocysts, are capable of infecting a vertebrate host. The potential infectivity of these sporozoites may be important as an alternate method of transmission.

The number of sporozoites contained in the salivary glands (33) and the number injected when the mosquito ingests a blood meal can be evaluated by artificial feeding experiments through membranes (49). If only one salivary gland lobe is infected with sporozoites, the probability of the lobe being emptied of its contents when the mosquito feeds is unknown. Likewise unknown is whether, depending on the number of sporozoites in the lobe, the mosquito would empty the entire contents in the first feeding probe or in multiple feedings. These data are important in reevaluating models to more accurately reflect the biological factors that play a role in transmission of plasmodia.

REFERENCES

(1) Ross, R. On some peculiar pigmented cells found in two mosquitoes fed on malarial blood. *Br Med J* ii:1786, 1897.

(2) Christophers, R. Insect vectors. Pp. 225–256 *in*: Boyd, M. F. (ed.), *Malariology*. Philadelphia: W. B. Saunders Co., 1949.

(3) Bray, R. S., and P. C. C. Garnham. Anopheles as vectors of animal malaria parasites. *Bull WHO* 31:143–147, 1964.

(4) Green, R. Observations on some factors influencing the infectivity of malarial gamete carriers in Malaya to *Anopheles maculatus*. *Bull Inst Med Research Federated Malay States* 5:1–41, 1929.

(5) Coatney, G. R., W. E. Collins, McW. Warren, and P. G. Contacos. *The Primate Malarias*. Washington, D.C.: U.S. Department of Health, Education, and Welfare, 1971.

(6) Warren, McW., W. E. Collins, G. M. Jeffrey, and B. B. Richardson. *Anopheles pseudopunctipennis*. Laboratory maintenance and malaria susceptibility of a strain from El Salvador. *Am J Trop Med Hyg* 29:503–506, 1980.

(7) Boyd, M. F., R. Christophers, and L. T. Coggeshall. Laboratory diagnosis of malaria infections. Pp. 155-204 *in*: Boyd, M. F. (ed.), *Malariology*. Philadelphia: W. B. Saunders Co., 1949.

(8) Das, P. K., R. Reuben, and C. P. Batra. Urban malaria and its vectors in Salem (Tamil Nadu): Natural and induced infection with human plasmodia in mosquitoes. *Indian J Med Res* 69:403–411, 1979.

(9) Bruce-Chwatt, L. J., C. Garrett-Jones, and B. Weitz. Ten years' study (1955-64) of host selection by anopheline mosquitoes. *Bull WHO* 35:405–439, 1966.

(10) Coluzzi, M. Heterogeneities of the malaria vectorial system in tropical Africa and their significance in malaria epidemiology and control. *Bull WHO* 62:107–113, 1984.

(11) Carpenter, S. J., and W. J. LaCosse. *Mosquitoes of North America*. Berkeley: University of California Press, 1955.

(12) Collins, W. E., McW. Warren, J. C. Skinner, and B. B. Sutton. Infectivity of two strains of *Plasmodium vivax* to *Anopheles albitarsis* mosquitoes from Colombia. *J Parasitol* 71:771–773, 1985.

(13) Warren, McW., W. E. Collins, B. B. Richardson, and J. C. Skinner. Morphological variants of *Anopheles albimanus* and susceptibility to *Plasmodium vivax* and *P. falciparum*. *Am J Trop Med Hyg* 26:607–611, 1977.

(14) Ramsdale, C. D., and M. Coluzzi. Studies on the infectivity of tropical African strains of *Plasmodium falciparum* to some southern European vectors of malaria. WHO/MAL/75:859:1–7. Geneva, 1975.

(15) Rutledge, L. C., D. J. Gould, and B. Tantichareon. Factors affecting the infection of anophelines with human malaria in Thailand. *Trans R Soc Trop Med Hyg* 63:613–619, 1969.

(16) World Health Organization. Malaria antigens associated with transmission-blocking immunity: Report of the eighth meeting of the scientific working group on the immunology of malaria. TDR/IMMAL/SWG(8)/85.3, 1985.

(17) Munesinghe, Y. D., K. N. Mendis, and R. Carter. Anti-gamete antibodies block transmission of human *vivax* malaria to mosquitoes. *Parasite Immunol* 8:231–238, 1986.

(18) Hawking, F., M. J. Worms, and K. Gammage. 24- and 48-hour cycles of malaria parasites in the blood; their purpose, production and control. *Trans R Soc Trop Med Hyg* 62:731–760, 1968.

(19) Jeffrey, G. M. Infectivity to mosquitoes of *Plasmodium vivax* and *Plasmodium falciparum* under various conditions. *Am J Trop Med Hyg* 9:315–320, 1960.

(20) Collins, W. E. Comparative infectivity of *Plasmodium falciparum* (Colombia strain) to *Anopheles quadrimaculatus* Say and *Anopheles albimanus* (Wied.). *Mosq News* 22:257–259, 1962.

(21) Collins, W. E., T. C. Orihel, P. G. Contacos, M. H. Jeter, and L. S. Gell. Some observations of the sporogonic cycle of *Plasmodium schwetzi*, *P. vivax* and *P. ovale* in five species of *Anopheles*. *J Protozool* 16:589–596, 1969.

(22) Collins, W. E., J. C. Skinner, McW. Warren, and B. Richardson. Studies on human malaria in *Aotus* monkeys. VII. Comparative infectivity of two strains of *Plasmodium vivax* to *Anopheles freeborni*, *A. maculatus*, and four strains of *A. albimanus*. *J Parasitol* 62:190–194, 1976.

(23) Collins, W. E., McW. Warren, J. C. Skinner, and B. B. Richardson. Studies on the West Pakistan strain of *Plasmodium vivax* in *Aotus* monkeys and anopheline mosquitoes. *J Parasitol* 66:780–785, 1980.

(24) Collins, W. E., McW. Warren, J. C. Skinner, A. Y. Huong, and P. Nguyen-Dinh. Observations on the infectivity of two strains of *Plasmodium vivax* from Vietnamese refugees to *Aotus* monkeys and anopheline mosquitoes. *J Parasitol* 69:689–695, 1983.

(25) Bruce-Chwatt, L. J. *Essential Malariology*. London: W. Heinemann Medical Books Ltd., 1980.

(26) Shute, P. G., and M. E. Maryon. *Laboratory Technique for the Study of Malaria*. London: J. & A. Churchill Ltd., 1960.

(27) Venters, D., M. Spencer, and S. H. Christian. Field and laboratory methods in malaria entomology. *Papua New Guinea Med J* 17:36–41, 1974.

(28) World Health Organization. *Manual on Practical Entomology in Malaria. Part II, Methods and Techniques*. Offset Publication No. 13. Geneva, 1975.

(29) Young, M. D., T. H. Stubbs, J. M. Ellis, R. W. Burgess, and D. E. Eyles. Studies on imported malarias: 4. The infectivity of malarias of foreign origin to anophelines of the southern United States. *Am J Hyg* 43:325–341, 1946.

(30) Brumpt, E. The human parasites of the genus *Plasmodium*. Pp. 65–121 in: Boyd, M. F. (ed.), *Malariology*. Philadelphia: W. B. Saunders Co., 1949.

(31) Huff, C. G. Life cycles of malaria parasites with special reference to the newer knowledge of pre-erythrocytic stages. Pp. 54–64 in: Boyd, M. F. (ed.), *Malariology*. Philadelphia: W. B. Saunders Co., 1949.

(32) Rutledge, L. C., R. A. Ward, and R. M. Buckwalter. *Plasmodium* spp.: Dispersion of malarial oocyst populations in anopheline and culicine mosquitoes. *Exp Parasitol* 34(1):132–141, 1973.

(33) Pringle, G. A quantitative study of naturally acquired malaria infections in *Anopheles gambiae* and *Anopheles funestus* in a highly malarious area of East Africa. *Trans R Soc Trop Med Hyg* 60(5):626–632, 1966.

(34) Sinden, R. E., and K. Strong. An ultrastructural study of the sporogonic development of *Plasmodium falciparum* in *Anopheles gambiae*. *Trans R Soc Trop Med Hyg* 72:477–491, 1978.

(35) Ramsey, J. M., R. L. Beaudoin, M. P. Bawden, and C. A. Espinal. Specific identification of *Plasmodium* sporozoites using an indirect fluorescent antibody method. *Trans R Soc Trop Med Hyg* 77:378–381, 1983.

(36) Burkot, T. R., F. Zavala, R. W. Gwadz, F. H. Collins, R. S. Nussenzweig, and D. R. Roberts. Identification of malaria-infected mosquitoes by a two-site enzyme-linked immunosorbent assay. *Am J Trop Med Hyg* 33:227–231, 1984.

(37) Zavala, F., R. W. Gwadz, F. H. Collins, R. S. Nussenzweig, and V. Nussenzweig. Monoclonal antibodies to circumsporozoite proteins identify the species of malaria parasite in infected mosquitoes. *Nature* 299:737–738, 1982.

(38) MacDonald, G. *The Epidemiology and Control of Malaria*. London: Oxford University Press, 1957.

(39) Molineaux, L., and G. Gramiccia. *The Garki Project. Research on the Epidemiology and Control of Malaria in the Sudan Savanna of West Africa*. Geneva: World Health Organization, 1980.

(40) Harwood, R. F., and M. T. James. *Entomology in Human and Animal Health*, 7th edition. New York: Macmillan Publ. Co., 1979.

(41) Ramsey, J. M., D. N. Bown, J. L. Aron, R. L. Beaudoin, and J. F. Méndez. Field trial in Chiapas, Mexico, of a rapid detection method for malaria in anopheline vectors with low infection rates. *Am J Trop Med Hyg* 35:234–238, 1986.

(42) Bosworth, A. B., I. Schneider, and J. E. Freier. Mass isolation of *Anopheles stephensi* salivary glands infected with malarial sporozoites. *J Parasitol* 61:769–772, 1975.

(43) Mack, S. R., J. P. Vanderberg, and R. Nawrot. Column separation of *Plasmodium berghei* sporozoites. *J Parasitol* 64:166–168, 1978.

(44) Moser, G., F. H. Brohn, H. D. Danforth, and R. S. Nussenzweig. Sporozoites of rodent and simian malaria, purified by anion exchangers, retain their immunogenicity and infectivity. *J Protozool* 25:119–124, 1978.

(45) Ozaki, L. S., R. W. Gwadz, and G. N. Godson. Simple centrifugation method for rapid separation of sporozoites from mosquitoes. *J Parasitol* 70:831–833, 1984.

(46) Pacheco, N. D., C. P. A. Strome, F. Mitchell, M. P. Bawden, and R. L. Beaudoin. Rapid, large-scale isolation of *Plasmodium berghei* sporozoites from infected mosquitoes. *J Parasitol* 65:414–417, 1979.

(47) Wood, D. E., L. L. Smrkovski, E. McConnell, N. D. Pacheco, and M. P. Bawden. The use of membrane screen filters in the isolation of *Plasmodium berghei* sporozoites from mosquitoes. *Bull WHO* 57(Suppl. 1):69–74, 1979.

(48) Walliker, D. An infection of *Plasmodium berghei* derived from sporozoites of a single oocyst. *Trans R Soc Trop Med Hyg* 66(4):543, 1972.

(49) Vanderberg, J. P. *Plasmodium berghei*: Quantitation of sporozoites injected by mosquitoes feeding on a rodent host. *Exp Parasitol* 42:169–181, 1977.

Chapter 7

DETECTION OF MALARIA PARASITES IN THE MOSQUITO BY IMMUNOLOGIC METHODS

Fidel Zavala

The sporozoite rate, that is, the prevalence of female anopheline mosquitoes with sporozoites in their salivary glands, is a very useful parameter for ascertaining the dynamics of malaria transmission in a given area. The sporozoite rate and the man-biting rate taken together provide an estimate of the number of potentially infective bites a person could expect to receive at the place and time the mosquitoes were collected (1, 2).

However, the sporozoite rate is extremely difficult to determine by microscopic techniques, which require that the salivary glands of freshly captured mosquitoes be removed and individually examined. This laborious and time-consuming procedure is seldom attempted, especially in areas of moderate to low malaria endemicity, where sporozoite rates are usually a fraction of a percent (3, 4). Thus, in many malarious regions of the world, even the primary vectors have not been conclusively identified. Furthermore, the lack of clear species-specific differences in sporozoite morphology severely restricts the utility of dissection-based determinations.

The sporozoite rate can serve as an indicator of the efficacy of control programs based on mass drug administration, use of biological or chemical insecticides, integrated pest management schemes, or the much-anticipated antimalaria vaccines. Given the large sums of money expended annually for the control of malaria, the lack of a coherent system or reliable technology for determining the effects of these programs is a serious deficiency.

The production of monoclonal antibodies specific for the principal surface antigen of the sporozoites of a number of different *Plasmodium* species (5) has made possible an immunologic procedure to detect sporozoites in infected mosquitoes (6). This procedure provides a rapid species-specific determination of both the presence and number of sporozoites in an infected mosquito. It can be performed on freshly caught or dried mosquitoes, because the antigen remains fully detectable for at least four months.

ANTIGENIC CHARACTERIZATION OF *PLASMODIUM* SPOROZOITES

Extensive studies on antisporozoite immunity directed towards the development of an antisporozoite vaccine have provided much information on the antigenic make-up of the sporozoite surface. By using monoclonal antibodies raised against sporozoites, the main surface antigen of the sporozoites has been identified. This protein, named the circumsporozoite (CS) protein, is found mainly on mature sporozoites and is uniformly distributed on their surface membrane (7). It is stage-specific to sporozoites, since it is not present on the blood stages of the parasite.

The CS protein is also a species-specific antigen. Most of the monoclonal antibodies raised against sporozoites of human (8), nonhuman primate (9), and rodent (10) malaria do not show significant cross-reactivity. Importantly, a species-specific CS protein of P. falciparum or P. vivax seems to be present in all isolates tested to date regardless of geographic origin (11). A monoclonal antibody (2A10) raised originally against P. falciparum sporozoites from Thailand recognizes sporozoites from isolates of that species that originated in Africa and Central and South America. The same ubiquity is characteristic of a monoclonal antibody specific for the CS protein of P. vivax (11).

Using monoclonal antibodies and recombinant DNA techniques, genes encoding the CS protein of the human malaria parasites P. falciparum (12, 13) and P. vivax (14, 15), as well as plasmodia causing monkey (16, 17) and rodent (18) malarias, have been cloned and the entire amino acid sequence elucidated. All these CS proteins share unusual antigenic and structural features. On the basis of sequence, charge densities, and secondary structure predictions, the CS proteins, which are formed by approximately 400 amino acids, can be divided into several domains. The most prominent is the central area formed by tandem repeats of 4 to 12 amino acids. This repeat domain represents 30% to 40% of the total protein, and its sequence varies greatly among the different species of plasmodia. In contrast, the flanking regions show areas of significant homology between different species.

The central repeat domain contains the main antigenic deteminants recognized by antisporozoite antibodies. The flanking regions seem to be much less immunogenic, but may play an important role in establishing antisporozoite immunity by sensitizing T lymphocytes (19).

The precise sequence of the antigenic determinants located in the repeat domain has been determined for the CS protein of several species. For example, the P. knowlesi CS protein contains 12 repeats of 12 amino acids each. Most of the monoclonal antibodies produced against this CS protein recognize a sequence of six to eight amino acids located within each repeat (20). In the case of P. falciparum, the repeat domain of the CS protein is formed by approximately 40 repeats of four amino acids. The antibodies recognize a sequence formed by 8 to 12 amino acids (21); therefore, two to three repeats of the four amino acids are needed to form an antigenic determinant, or epitope.

Based on the structure of the repeat domain of the CS protein, it can be easily inferred that each CS protein molecule has the capacity to bind simultaneously several antibodies of the same specificity. In fact, studies undertaken before the amino acid sequence was elucidated had already detected the polyvalent character of the CS proteins and the presence of repeated epitopes (22).

THE TWO-SITE IMMUNOASSAY

Because the CS protein can bind more than one antibody simultaneously, a two-site assay for its detection and quantification was designed.

Monoclonal antibodies that recognize the repeated epitopes are bound to wells on plastic (polyvinylchloride) microtiter plates as the result of charge interactions between the protein and the plastic surface. This binding is obtained by incubating the wells with the monoclonal antibody solution for a period of 4 to 12 hours and then washing the wells to discard all the unbound antibodies. At this stage, the immobilized antibodies are firmly attached to the plastic and retain their antigen-binding properties (Figure 7.1A).

Since the antibodies may not totally saturate the plastic, it is necessary to incubate the wells with an unrelated protein, such as casein or albumin (Figure 7.1B). This step ensures that the reagents to be added subsequently will bind only through specific interactions and not by passive absorption to the plastic.

The sample containing the antigen can then be placed in each well and incubated for two hours or longer, during which time the antigen will bind to the immobilized antibody (Figure 7.1C). The extent of this binding will depend on the antigen concentration, amount of immobilized antibody, and strength of the antigen-antibody interaction (affinity).

After incubation with the antigen is completed, the wells are washed to get rid of any unbound antigen and then incubated again with a solution containing labeled antibody. Antigen bound to the immobilized antibody still has free antigenic determinants available for the binding of the labeled antibody (Figure 7.1D). The antibody can be labeled with ^{125}I (immunoradiometric assay or IRMA) or with peroxidase (enzyme-linked immunosorbent assay or ELISA). After incubation with the radio-labeled antibody (two-site IRMA), the wells are washed and each well is placed in a gamma counter. The amount of radioactivity detected reflects the amount of antibody bound. If the antibody was labeled with an enzyme (two-site ELISA), a substrate is added to each well to reveal the reaction. The enzymatic reaction induces a color change in the substrate solution, which can be measured in an ELISA reader.

Thus, the CS protein assay can be performed as a two-site IRMA or a two-site ELISA (23). Both assays are based in the same principle and differ only in the method of labeling the antibody and reading the reaction. A comparison of the specificity and sensitivity of the two assays shows that they give essentially the same results (Figure 7.2). The advantage of the ELISA is that the enzyme-labeled antibodies have a considerably longer shelf-life. Furthermore, in some countries it is difficult to obtain radioactive reagents and to dispose of them after use. At the present time, adaptations of the ELISA have been described for the detection of P. falciparum (24, 25) and also P. vivax sporozoites (25, 26).

Initial experiments using a known quantity of sporozoites showed that this assay could detect protein reflecting less than 50 sporozoites. This level of sensitivity ensured that practically all experimentally infected mosquitoes would be detected by the assay, since Anopheles usually harbor several hundreds or thousands of sporozoites in their salivary glands.

In testing this methodology, the whole body of an infected mosquito was individually "processed." A mosquito extract is obtained by grinding, with a sealed Pasteur pipette, mosquitoes suspended in 30 microliters of phosphate-buffered saline solution (PBS) containing 1% bovine serum albumin (BSA) and 0.5% Nonidet P-40 (NP-40) as a detergent. The addition of detergent is necessary to ensure solubilization of the CS protein; alternately, sonication may be used. After grinding each mosquito (a process that takes 5 to 10 seconds), additional PBS-BSA is added to dilute the detergent, which at high concentrations can affect the sensitivity of the assay. An aliquot of this extract is then used to perform the test.

The studies performed with experimentally infected mosquitoes (6) provided some important basic information.

1. The assay was not only sensitive enough to detect infection in the mosquitoes, but also correctly identified the species of the plasmodia to which the sporozoites belonged.

2. The antigenic activity of the CS protein was fully conserved in dead mosquitoes that had been maintained for several weeks or months in a dry environment. This property of the sporozoite antigen facilitates considerably the central-laboratory screening of infected mosquitoes from endemic areas.

3. Since the extent of the binding of the labeled antibody depended on the amount of antigen present, this assay was also quantitative. As a consequence, it allowed an estimation of the number of sporozoites present in each mosquito (sporozoite load).

4. Since only a fraction of the extract of each mosquito is used in each assay, a single mosquito can be probed for the presence of several species of sporozoites using monoclonal antibodies against different species. The assay therefore detects the presence of mixed infections, as well as the capacity of a given vector to become infected with different plasmodia species.

5. It was also found that pools of 20 mosquitoes could be assayed without losing the specificity or reducing significantly the sensitivity of the assay. This may be particularly important in those endemic areas where the sporozoite rates are very low.

DETECTION OF NATURALLY INFECTED MOSQUITOES

In order to definitively establish the usefulness of this assay, a field trial was conducted in The Gambia, West Africa (27). A total of 2,569 *Anopheles gambiae* (sibling species) and *An. arabiensis* were caught during the months of October and November of 1982. Half of these mosquitoes were dissected and their salivary glands examined by microscopy to determine the sporozoite infection rate. The remaining mosquitoes were killed, stored in a dry environment, and subsequently processed by immunoassay. The sporozoite rate obtained by microscopic examination was 5.5%, while the rate obtained by the immunoassay was 7.3%.

By constructing a standard curve based on an extract containing a known number of sporozoites, it was possible to estimate the sporozoite load of each mosquito. The results showed that more than 35% of the *Anopheles* had between 500 and 4,000 sporozoites; the maximum load was approximately 100,000. These results are very similar to those obtained when sporozoites present in the salivary glands of mosquitoes captured in Tanzania were counted under the microscope.

The results of this first field trial proved that the assay does in fact have the sensitivity and specificity to detect naturally infected mosquitoes and therefore could become a useful tool for entomological and epidemiological investigations.

Similar studies have recently been reported. In Papua New Guinea, a comparison was made between the sporozoite rate obtained with a two-site ELISA and the results of microscopic examination of mosquito salivary glands (29). The study encompassed four villages from an area of Papua New Guinea of high malaria endemicity. The principal malaria vectors in this area are members of the *Anopheles punc-*

tulatus complex: *An. farauti*, *An. koliensis*, and *An. punctulatus*. Immunoassay was used to test 669 specimens of this complex, and a similar number were examined microscopically. The sporozoite rate determined by microscopy was 4.0%, while immunoassay gave a rate of 3.4%, a difference that was not statistically significant. Mosquitoes of all the different species were shown to be positive for *P. vivax* (1.49%) and for *P. falciparum* (1.94%) by immunoassay.

In the Amazon region of Brazil, 10,000 mosquitoes were examined (*25*). This study compared the results obtained by the IRMA and the ELISA tests and found that both assays gave essentially the same results. *P. vivax* infections were found in 16.7% to 1% of the mosquitoes and *P. falciparum* in 8.3% to 0.2%, with sporozoite rates varying greatly between different localities. Interestingly, *P. falciparum* infections were restricted to *An. darlingi* and *An. oswaldi*, while *P. vivax* infections were found in several additional mosquito species (*An. triannulatus*, *An. albitarsis*, and *An. nuneztovari*) (*25*).

Other studies have obtained rates with the immunoassay that were as much as two times higher than those obtained by microscopic examination of the salivary glands (*30*). This apparent discrepancy seems to be caused in part by the lower sensitivity of microscopic examination, which may fail to detect infected salivary glands that have low sporozoite loads (*31*).

Nonetheless, it is important to stress that the results obtained with the immunoassay, which uses mosquito extracts, cannot necessarily be equated to salivary gland sporozoite rates, since the assay detects CS antigen present in the entire mosquito and does not differentiate between salivary gland, hemocoel, or oocyst sporozoites. It has, in fact, been found that the CS antigen appears in the later stages of development of oocysts, before migration of the sporozoites to the salivary glands. In assays performed with whole specimens of naturally infected mosquitoes captured in Burkina Faso, it was found that 10% of the positive *Anopheles* contained the CS antigen only in the abdomens (*30*). Furthermore, studies on mosquitoes experimentally infected with *P. cynomolgi* (*32*) and *P. falciparum* (*30*) have revealed the presence of detectable CS protein in their midguts 10 days after an infective meal, that is, 24 to 48 hours before the sporozoites reach the salivary glands. Overestimation of the number of "infective" mosquitoes, caused by the presence of antigen in the abdomen, can be eliminated by processing only the thorax, which can easily be isolated from the remainder of the mosquito's body.

A recent study performed in Burkina Faso describes another factor that may also account for the observed difference of results obtained by microscopy and immunoassay. When thoraxes and salivary glands from the same mosquitoes were analyzed by both methods, it was found that in one particular village a considerable percentage (43%) of positive mosquitoes had detectable CS antigen only in their thoraxes and not in their salivary glands. The failure of sporozoites to migrate to the salivary glands seemed to be intrinsic to these mosquitoes, since keeping them alive under laboratory conditions for several days prior to the assay did not result in an increased percentage of salivary gland infections (*31*). In this regard, pertinent earlier observations also exist indicating that some *Anopheles* species are capable of supporting development of oocyst sporozoites that subsequently cannot migrate to the salivary glands (*33, 34*).

Therefore, to incriminate as malaria vectors any new, additional species of *Anopheles* found to be positive by the immunoassay, evidence of the presence of CS antigen and/or sporozoites in the salivary glands would be required. Such proof could be obtained by experimentally infecting mosquitoes by feeding them on "in vitro" blood cultures containing sexual forms or on infected animals.

CONCLUSION

The experimental data as well as the results of field trials clearly indicate that an immunoassay that detects the CS protein can have considerable value for epidemiological and entomological studies.

Because the assay can be done rapidly and on dried mosquitoes, it permits basic studies of malaria transmission that were previously beyond the resources of most malaria control programs. An important benefit will be the determination of the relative importance of different anopheline species and subspecies in the transmission of various human malaria parasites, particularly in areas of mesoendemic, hypoendemic, or unstable malaria. This technique will also make it possible to determine the relationship between inoculation rates and incidence, the two direct measures of malaria transmission. The often-recorded discrepancy between entomological inoculation rates and incidence in endemic areas suggests that sporozoite load may be an important factor in the efficacy of the mosquito vector of malaria.

Vector infection rates, unlike malaria incidence in humans, should be immediately responsive to changes in the level of malaria transmission. The application of this immunoassay to epidemiological analyses in endemic areas should provide information of immediate use for ongoing or planned malaria control programs.

REFERENCES

(1) MacDonald, G. The analysis of the sporozoite rate. *Trop Dis Bull* 49:569–585, 1952.

(2) MacDonald, G. *The Epidemiology and Control of Malaria*. London: Oxford University Press, 1957.

(3) Pampana, E. *A Textbook of Malaria Eradication*. London: Oxford University Press, 1963.

(4) Warren, M., J. Mason, and J. Hobbs. Natural infections of *Anopheles albimanus* with *Plasmodium* in a small malaria focus. *Am J Trop Med Hyg* 24:545–546, 1975.

(5) Nussenzweig, V., and R. S. Nussenzweig. Circumsporozoite proteins of malaria parasites. *Cell* 42:401–403, 1985.

(6) Zavala, F., R. W. Gwadz, F. H. Collins, R. S. Nussenzweig, and V. Nussenzweig. Monoclonal antibodies to circumsporozoite proteins identify the species of malaria parasite in infected mosquitoes. *Nature* 299:737–738, 1982.

(7) Aikawa, M., N. Yoshida, R. S. Nussenzweig, and V. Nussenzweig. The protective antigen of malarial sporozoitic *Plasmodium berghei* is a differentiation antigen. *J Immunol* 126:2494–2495, 1981.

(8) Nardin, E. H., V. Nussenzweig, R. S. Nussenzweig, W. E. Collins, K. T. Harinasuta, P. Tapchaisri, and Y. Chomcharn. Circumsporozoite (CS) proteins of human malaria parasites *Plasmodium falciparum* and *Plasmodium vivax*. *J Exp Med* 156:20–30, 1982.

(9) Cochrane, A. H., F. Santoro, V. Nussenzweig, R. W. Gwadz, and R. S. Nussenzweig. Monoclonal antibodies identify the protective antigens of sporozoites of *Plasmodium knowlesi*. *Proc Natl Acad Sci USA* 79:5651–5655, 1982.

(10) Yoshida, N., R. S. Nussenzweig, P. Potocnjak, V. Nussenzweig, and M. Aikawa. Hybridoma produces protective antibodies against the sporozoite stage of malaria parasite. *Science* 207:71–73, 1980.

(11) Zavala, F., A. Masuda, P. M. Graves, V. Nussenzweig, and R. S. Nussenzweig. Ubiquity of the repetitive epitope of the CS protein in different isolates of human malaria parasites. *J Immunol* 135:1–4, 1985.

(12) Dame, J. B., J. L. Williams, T. F. McCutchan, J. L. Weber, R. A. Wirtz, W. T. Hockmeyer, W. L. Maloy, J. D. Haynes, I. Schneider, D. Roberts, G. S. Sanders, E. P. Reddy, C. L. Diggs, and L. H. Miller. Structure of the gene encoding the immunodominant surface antigen on the sporozoite of the human malaria parasite *Plasmodium falciparum*. *Science* 225:593–599, 1984.

(13) Enea, V., J. Ellis, F. Zavala, D. E. Arnot, A. Asavanich, A. Masuda, I. Quakyi, and R. S. Nussenzweig. DNA cloning of *Plasmodium falciparum* circumsporozoite gene: Amino acid sequence of repetitive epitope. *Science* 225:628–630, 1984.

(14) Arnot, D. E., J. W. Barnwell, J. P. Tam, V. Nussenzweig, R. S. Nussenzweig, and V. Enea. Circumsporozoite protein of *Plasmodium vivax*: Gene cloning and characterization of the immunodominant epitope. *Science* 230:815–818, 1985.

(15) McCutchan, T. F., A. A. Lal, V. de la Cruz, L. H. Miller, W. L. Maloy, Y. Charoenvit, R. L. Beaudoin, P. Guerry, R. Wistar, Jr., S. L. Hoffman, W. T. Hockmeyer, W. E. Collins, and D. Wirth. Sequence of the immunodominant epitope for the surface protein on sporozoites of *Plasmodium vivax*. *Science* 230:1381–1383, 1985.

(16) Godson, G. N., J. Ellis, P. Svec, D. H. Schlesinger, and V. Nussenzweig. Identification and chemical synthesis of an epitope of the *Plasmodium knowlesi* circumsporozoite protein. Evidence for its tandemly repeated nature. *Nature* 305:29–33, 1983.

(17) Galinski, M. R., D. E. Arnot, A. H. Cochrane, J. W. Barnwell, R. S. Nussenzweig, and V. Enea. The circumsporozoite gene of the *Plasmodium cynomolgi* complex. *Cell* 48(2):311–320, 1987.

(18) Eichinger, D. J., D. E. Arnot, J. P. Tam, V. Nussenzweig, and V. Enea. The circumsporozoite protein of *P. berghei*: Gene cloning and identification of the immunodominant epitope. *Molec Cell Biol* 6:3965–3972, 1986.

(19) Good, M. F., J. A. Berzofsky, W. L. Maloy, Y. Hayashi, N. Fujii, W. T. Hockmeyer, and L. H. Miller. Genetic control of the immune response in mice to a *Plasmodium falciparum* sporozoite vaccine: Widespread nonresponsiveness to single malaria T epitope in highly repetitive vaccine. *J Exp Med* 164:655–661, 1986.

(20) Schlesinger, D. H., A. H. Cochrane, R. W. Gwadz, G. N. Godson, R. Melton, R. S. Nussenzweig, and V. Nussenzweig. Structure of an immunodominant epitope of the circumsporozoite surface protein of *Plasmodium knowlesi*. *Biochemistry* 23:5665–5670, 1984.

(21) Zavala, F., J. P. Tam, M. R. Hollingdale, A. H. Cochrane, I. Quakyi, R. S. Nussenzweig, and V. Nussenzweig. Rationale for development of a synthetic vaccine against *Plasmodium falciparum* malaria. *Science* 228:1436–1440, 1985.

(22) Zavala, F., A. H. Cochrane, E. H. Nardin, R. S. Nussenzweig, and V. Nussenzweig. Circumsporozoite proteins of malaria parasites contain a single immunodominant region with two or more identical epitopes. *J Exp Med* 157:1947–1957, 1983.

(23) Burkot, T. R., F. Zavala, R. W. Gwadz, F. H. Collins, R. S. Nussenzweig, and D. R. Roberts. Identification of malaria infected mosquitoes by a two-site enzyme-linked immunosorbent assay. *Am J Trop Med Hyg* 33:227–231, 1984.

(24) Burkot, T. R., J. L. Williams, and I. Schneider. Identification of *Plasmodium falciparum* infected mosquitoes by a double antibody enzyme-linked immunosorbent assay. *Am J Trop Med Hyg* 33:783–788, 1984.

(25) de Arruda, M., M. B. Cavalho, R. S. Nussenzweig, M. Maracic, A. W. Ferreira, and A. H. Cochrane. Potential vectors of malaria and their different susceptibility to *P. falciparum* and *P. vivax* in Northern Brazil identified by immunoassay. *Am J Trop Med Hyg* 35:873–881, 1986.

(26) Wirtz, R. A., T. R. Burkot, R. G. Andre, R. Rosenberg, W. E. Collins, and D. R. Roberts. Identification of *Plasmodium vivax* sporozoites in mosquitoes using an enzyme-linked immunosorbent assay. *Am J Trop Med Hyg* 34:1049–1054, 1985.

(27) Collins, F. H., F. Zavala, P. M. Graves, A. H. Cochrane, R. W. Gwadz, J. Akoh, and R. S. Nussenzweig. First field trial of an immunoradiometric assay for the detection of malaria sporozoites in mosquitoes. *Am J Trop Med Hyg* 33:538–543, 1984.

(28) Pringle, G. A quantitative study of naturally acquired malaria infections in *Anopheles gambiae* and *Anopheles funestus* in a highly malarious area of East Africa. *Trans R Soc Trop Med Hyg* 60:626–632, 1966.

(29) Wirtz, R. A., T. R. Burkot, P. M. Graves, and R. G. Andre. Field evaluation of enzyme-linked immunosorbent assays (ELISAs) for *P. falciparum* or *P. vivax* sporozoites in mosquitoes from Papua New Guinea. *J Med Entomol* 24:433–437, 1987.

(30) Esposito, F., S. Lombardi, Y. T. Toure, F. Zavala, and M. Coluzzi. Field observations on the use of antisporozoite monoclonal antibodies for determination of infection rates in malaria vectors. *Parassitologia* 28:68–77, 1986.

(31) Lombardi, S., F. Esposito, F. Zavala, L. Lamizana, P. Rossi, G. Sabatinelli, R. S. Nussenzweig, and M. Coluzzi. Detection and anatomical localization of *Plasmodium falciparum* circumsporozoite protein and sporozoites in the Afrotropical malaria vector *Anopheles gambiae* S. L., 1986. *Am J Trop Med Hyg* 37:491–494, 1987.

(32) Collins, F. C., R. W. Gwadz, L. C. Koontz, F. Zavala, and R. S. Nussenzweig. Laboratory assessment of a species-specific radioimmunoassay for the detection of malaria sporozoites in mosquitoes (Diptera: Culicidae). *J Med Entomol* 22:121–129, 1985.

(33) Coatney, G. R., W. E. Collins, McW. Warren, and P. G. Contacos. *The Primate Malarias*. Washington, D.C.: U.S. Department of Health, Education, and Welfare, 1971.

(34) Rosenberg, R. Inability of *Plasmodium knowlesi* sporozoites to invade *Anopheles freeborni* salivary glands. *Am J Trop Med Hyg* 34:687–691, 1985.

Chapter 8

IMMUNODIAGNOSIS OF MALARIA

Antonio Walter Ferreira

A patient's history and clinical examination often are insufficient to make an etiologic diagnosis of malaria, and it then becomes necessary to resort to direct observation of the parasite in the host, the most specific method for confirming the diagnosis. Unfortunately, this is not the ideal method, given the low sensitivity, the expense, and the technical complexity of the techniques used, and/or the lack of specialized personnel.

Although immunologic techniques are useful for confirming or ruling out a diagnosis and for the ongoing surveillance of the patient, no single test is available that determines the presence or absence of malaria. This is because the immune response is influenced by several of the host's characteristics and occurs against antigenic determinants often common to parasites of a different genus and species. There are two important parameters in calibrating a serologic test: sensitivity and specificity. Both will determine the diagnostic test's validity.

The results of a serologic examination may be: a) true positives (TP), if those testing positive have or have had the infection; b) false positives (FP), if the individuals test positive but have never been exposed to the infection; c) true negatives (TN), if the individuals test negative and have never had the infection; and d) false negatives (FN), if they test negative even though they have or have had the infection. Sensitivity is defined as the number of true positive (TP) results multiplied by 100 and divided by the sum of true positives plus false negatives (TP + FN). Specificity is obtained by multiplying the number of true negatives (TN) by 100 and dividing this by the sum of true negatives plus false positives (TN + FP) (Table 8.1).

Another important factor is the serologic test's repeatability. This can be defined as obtaining concordant results when the test is conducted by different persons in different places. Calibration of the test, rigorous quality control of the reagents, appropriate training of technical personnel, and the use of standard reagents and sera are necessary conditions for repeating a serologic test. When the true positive or negative diagnosis is replaced by the results of a reference test, it must be taken into account that sensitivity and specificity may vary according to the disease's prevalence.

When specific quantitative serologic tests are conducted in a population testing true positive and in another with a true negative diagnosis, it is observed that serologic reactivity may be expressed in titer frequency distribution curves. As seen in Figure 8.1, the titer frequency distribution curves are superimposed for persons with malarial antibodies (a) and those lacking them (b) using the indirect hemagglutination technique. If the titer 1:4 is established as the lower limit, the test's sensitivity is increased, but its specificity is reduced. If the titer 1:16 is established as the lower limit, the specificity increases, but the sensitivity is reduced. If 1:8 is taken as the

Table 8.1. Binary combination to determine the parameters of a serologic test when the diagnosis is certain (TP = true positives, FP = false positives, FN = false negatives, TN = true negatives).

Test result	Presence of malaria		
	Yes	No	
Positive	TP	FP	$Sensitivity = \dfrac{TP \times 100}{(TP + FN)}$
Negative	FN	TN	$Specificity = \dfrac{TN \times 100}{(TN + FP)}$

lower-limit titer, the maximum sensitivity and specificity is obtained. In the case of malaria, it is possible to work with a variable lower limit depending on the tests' objectives. To rule out the disease, a test of the highest sensitivity is required (lower limit = 1:4), while for a clinical diagnosis it is necessary to conduct a test of the highest specificity (lower limit = 1:16). Based on this, it can be concluded that serologic test results merely have a predictive value, that is, the probability that when the test is positive the infection or disease is or has been present. When test results are negative, there is little or no probability that the individual is or has been infected.

A predictive value depends on the test's sensitivity and specificity and on the disease's prevalence in the population under study. The more prevalent the disease is, the greater will be the predictive value of a positive result; the less prevalent the disease is, the greater will be the predictive value of a negative result. Thus, the concept of predictive value may be applied to both positive and negative results (1).

The predictive value of a positive test, or positive predictive value (PPV), is defined as the probability that a person testing positive has or has had a malarial infection. The PPV is obtained by dividing the number of true positive samples by the total positive samples, including the false positives (PPV = TP/TP + FP). The predictive value of a negative test, or negative predictive value (NPV), is defined as the probability that a person testing negative does not have or has not had a malarial infection. The NPV is obtained by dividing the number of true negative samples by the total number of negative samples, including the false negatives (NPV = TN/TN + FN). Tables 8.2 and 8.3 show examples of the predictive value of a positive or negative test in populations with different malarial prevalences.

HUMORAL IMMUNE RESPONSE IN MALARIAL INFECTION

During the cycle of plasmodia in the vertebrate host, antigenic stimulation causes the formation of antibody globulins of varying specificity. Although this immune response makes immunodiagnosis possible, most of these immunoglobulins do not act against antigenic components of the plasmodia, but rather are heterophil antibodies or autoantibodies which act against the red blood cells, lymphocytes, the complement, the rheumatoid factor, and antinuclear factors. This nonspecific reactivity can be explained by the polyclonal activation of the B lymphocytes due to the

Table 8.2. Predictive value of a positive test with 95% sensitivity and 85% specificity in populations with different prevalences (PPV = TP/TP + FP) where TP = prevalance × sensitivity and FP = population lacking antibodies × 1−specificity).

	Prevalence	
Population	1%	5%
a) Population surveyed	10,000	10,000
b) Population with malarial antibodies	100	500
c) Population without malarial antibodies	9,900	9,500
d) True positive samples (TP) (b × 0.95)	95	475
e) False positive samples (FP) (c × 1 − 0.85)	1,485	1,425
f) Total positive samples (d + e)	1,580	1,900
Positive predictive value (PPV)(d/f)	$\dfrac{95}{1,580} = 6\%$	$\dfrac{475}{1,900} = 25\%$

Table 8.3. Predictive value of a negative test with 95% sensitivity and 85% specificity in populations with different prevalences (NPV = TN/TN + FN, where FN = persons without antibodies × specificity and FN = persons with the infection × 1−sensitivity).

	Prevalence	
Population	1%	5%
a) Population surveyed	10,000	10,000
b) Population with malarial antibodies	100	500
c) Population without malarial antibodies	9,900	9,500
d) True negative samples (TN) (c × 0.85)	8,415	8,075
e) False negative samples (FN) (b × 1 − 0.95)	5	25
f) Total negative samples (d + e)	8,420	8,100
Negative predictive value (NPV)(d/f)	$\dfrac{8,415}{8,420} = 99.9\%$	$\dfrac{8,075}{8,100} = 99.6\%$

mitogenic action of soluble plasmodia antigens. Several experimental studies suggest the presence of a dialyzable plasmodial mitogenic substance, stable at 56°C and destroyed at 100°C, which can induce polyclonal activation of the B lymphocytes, probably by means of T lymphocytes or accessory cells. Only a small portion of these immunoglobulins are specific antibodies against plasmodia antigens and an even smaller part of these are antibodies related to the host's functional immunity (2).

NONPROTECTIVE SPECIFIC IMMUNOGLOBULINS

After the first week of infection, immunoglobulins, which react with plasmodia antigens, are detected. The IgG and IgM antibodies remain in the infected host's circulation for long periods. Even though they have little correlation with the patient's clinical signs and symptoms, detection of these antibodies can help in the diagnosis, and it is also useful for epidemiological studies on prevalence and frequency.

Although the antibodies against the plasmodia are specific with regard to genus, cross reactivity between the different species is not complete and, depending on the test used, negative heterologous reactions may be observed. Therefore, to increase sensitivity and to determine the infection's prevalence, it is desirable to use the species of plasmodia which predominate in the study population as antigen for the serologic tests (3).

PROTECTIVE IMMUNOGLOBULINS

The protective immunoglobulins act against the sporozoites and the asexual erythrocytic forms. The importance of antibodies in immunity during the erythrocytic stage was determined through passive transfer of immune serum, suppression of the antibodies with anti-μ chain serum, monoclonal antibodies, or experimental immunization. In general, passive immunization is more efficient with sera from donors who have had several infections. The protective activity is related to the presence of IgG and IgM antibodies, and is usually more efficient when both are present. The antisporozoite antibodies, evaluated in serologic tests, play an important role in malarial immunity. The protection acquired is species and stage specific against the geographic variants of the same species.

In highly endemic areas, malarial immunity is acquired slowly, after long periods of exposure to the infection (4). In such areas, older people have a high degree of immunity and clinical malaria is infrequent, with a sterile immunity being observed very rarely (5). The newborn are usually protected during the early months of life by maternal antibodies. The decline in these antibodies makes children susceptible. With age, individual resistance to malaria increases and the parasites' reproduction usually declines (6). In general, immunity is acquired during adolescence in endemic areas and it often is related to periods of parasitic latency in the peripheral blood (7). Such immunity usually disappears when there is no repeated exposure to the infection.

IMMUNODIAGNOSIS OF MALARIA

Immunodiagnosis of malaria includes methods that evaluate the host's humoral and cellular immunity. The method followed should be sufficiently sensitive, specific, and repeatable to detect infections with low parasitemia, to differentiate previous infections from current infections and the initial infection from recurrences and reinfections, and to determine the degree of functional immunity. In many countries microscopic blood examinations (thick blood film) of febrile cases are conducted to measure the rate of patent parasitemias per 1,000 inhabitants and thus to be able to reach decisions concerning prevention and control programs. However, in endemic areas not everybody with malaria develops fever. Microscopic examination for parasites merely indicates the presence or absence of patent parasitemia at the time of the examination, which may be affected by the use of antimalarial drugs and by the host's immune status. Moreover, spleen measurement is used on a lesser scale because changes in the spleen index may be the result of other infectious processes unrelated to malaria.

Among existing immunologic techniques, serologic methods are useful in both endemic and nonendemic areas. In areas where malaria is or has been endemic, serologic methods are useful for: a) measuring malaria's endemicity; b) verifying the presence or absence of malarial infections; c) determining malarial areas; d) detecting seasonal changes in transmission; e) investigating the reintroduction of malaria in areas with control programs; and f) evaluating antimalarial activities (6, 8).

In areas where malaria is not endemic, serologic methods are useful for: a) screening blood donors; b) elucidating undetermined clinical cases; c) evaluating treatments; d) diagnosing febrile cases testing negative for parasites; e) detecting malaria in individuals returning from endemic areas; and f) detecting individuals with latent forms of the disease (mainly those infected by *P. vivax* and *P. malariae*) (6, 8).

SEROLOGIC TESTS FOR DIAGNOSING HUMAN MALARIA

INDIRECT IMMUNOFLUORESCENCE TEST (IIF)

This is considered a reference test in malaria serodiagnosis and seroepidemiology, and was originally used to detect antibodies in the sera of volunteers infected by *P. vivax* and *P. cynomolgi* (9). Using this same technique it was possible to determine the titers of antibodies in serum and to follow their production course (10). However, the specificity of this technique was not high, since there were cross reactions among the plasmodia (11).

Initial studies of the IIF test were made by using glass slides prepared with blood smears obtained from infected persons or nonhuman primates as a source of antigen. The low numbers of parasites per microscopic field led researchers to use the thick blood film technique with erythrocytes that had been washed with physiological salt solution (12). This method improved the test's sensitivity and specificity. Use of an autochthonous antigen gives the IIF test an advantage over others for which antigenic extracts or metabolic products are used (13). Moreover, many authors have reported contradictory results when antigens of plasmodia not related to human malaria have been used. It must be taken into account that the choice of an antigen depends on the test's objectives, since homologous antigens generally detect antibody titers at higher levels than heterologous antigens and also provide retrospective information on the population. Thus, simultaneous use of the antigens of plasmodia that cause human malaria makes it possible to differentiate the causative agents, even in the absence of parasitemia. The use of multispecific antigens increases the test's sensitivity, to the detriment of specificity, for which reason they should be used only to classify serum samples (14). Blood from individuals having an active primary infection may be used as a source of antigen. Although less accessible, there are two other possible sources of antigen—infections induced in nonhuman primates and continuous culture *in vitro* (15). In the first instance, *Aotus trivirgatus* and *Saimiri sciureus* monkeys are the species chosen for experimental infection by *P. falciparum* and *P. vivax*. Nevertheless, maintenance of animal facilities for these species is not justified merely for the purpose of obtaining antigen. In the case of *P. falciparum*, adaptation and development *in vitro* provide very appropriate antigens for serologic tests (16). When antigens from cultured whole parasitized erythrocytes were used to detect IgM antibodies in individuals living in endemic areas, the results indicated that the reaction was more sensitive, specific, and repeatable than the results from antigens obtained from the blood of infected persons (17). It was felt that conservation of the parasitic antigens present in the erythrocyte's membrane, conservation of soluble antigens of the parasite, and the uniformity of the parasites' degree of maturity were important factors in improving the test. Moreover, it was possible to correlate the concentration of IgM antibodies with the infections under way. Thus the IIF test is a useful instrument for clinical follow-up in endemic areas. Since the use of schizonts as antigen increases the IIF test's sensitivity, it is necessary to prepare antigens with the greatest possible proportion of mature schizonts.

Given the discrepancies among results obtained in various laboratories, several attempts have been made to standardize the IIF test. The World Health Organization (WHO) invited 12 laboratories to conduct an experiment on standardization of IIF tests and of passive hemagglutination (18). Each laboratory received slides prepared by a reference laboratory containing 5 to 10 parasites of *P. falciparum*, prepared from *in vitro* culture, per microscopic field. Lyophilized sera or plasmas with known titers were provided to obtain a negative and a positive anti-*P. falciparum*, anti-*P. vivax*, anti-*P. ovale*, and anti-*P. malariae* control. Also provided were anti-IgG (gamma chain) and anti-IgM (human antiglobulins) fluorescent conjugates with well-defined physical, chemical, and immunologic characteristics, and sensitized erythrocytes in suspension. Some laboratories used their own reagents.

Observations regarding the IIF test were as follows: a) better results were obtained with the reference laboratory plates than with those prepared by the participating laboratories; b) the reference conjugates were better than those prepared in the laboratories; and c) cross reactions were observed among the various plasmodium species studied.

WHO's work led to the conclusion that standardized production of reagents by specialized laboratories is superior to the small-scale production of some of the laboratories that took part in the study. This is easily explained by the rigorous quality control of reagents in reference laboratories so that the IIF test will have the greatest sensitivity, specificity, and repeatability.

To achieve an optimum IIF test for *P. falciparum*, the following variables must be taken into account (19): a) the source of antigen (proportion of schizonts); b) the preparation and conservation of antigens on slides; c) the diluent of the sera; and d) the quality of the microscope and source of UV illumination. The trials conducted indicate that:

a) the antigen obtained from cultures is superior to that obtained from infected hosts;

b) the dilution of sera in a phosphate-buffered saline solution containing 1% Tween 80 improves the test's sensitivity;

c) the techniques of stabilizing the slides in a desiccator containing silica gel and fixing with frozen acetone brought better results than the other techniques;

d) the slides with the antigenic suspension can be kept with a desiccant and vacuum-packed for long periods at room temperature without loss of immunologic activity; and

e) the geometric mean of the reciprocal of the titers of the sera from noninfected persons was always less than 20.

In longitudinal studies, the results of the IIF test showed that the antibodies are detected days after the parasitemia becomes patent and that the titers increase quickly, peaking after four to six weeks and gradually dropping when the antigenic stimulus stops immediately after the parasitological cure.

The IgM antibodies are usually the first to disappear from the bloodstream. The IgG antibodies' persistence depends on the infection's duration and intensity and the frequency of exposure to the specific antigen. In relapses there is an increase in the titers, which remain high during the parasitic latency. In endemic areas, the IIF test meets the minimum requirements for malarial serology and has been tested in several countries in population surveys.

The IIF test is also now used to find antisporozoite (20) and antimerozoite (21) antibodies, to evaluate an individual's immunity (22), and to determine malaria transmission levels (23).

IMMUNOENZYMATIC TEST

With whole parasites as antigen. The idea of conjugating the immunoglobulins with enzymes opened up new possibilities for immunodiagnosis. The initial steps in this field made it possible to link alkaline phosphatase to antibodies (24). Although they were satisfactory, results varied greatly. Moreover, when peroxidase was used to label the antibodies, the results were excellent. The preparations were stable and permanent and could be observed with an ordinary microscope (25).

When the indirect immunoperoxidase (IIP) test was used to investigate anti-plasmodium antibodies in blood smears fixed on plates, it was concluded that there were no significant differences between results obtained with the IIP and the IIF (26).

With soluble antigens. A significant advance in the development of serology was standardization of the enzyme-linked immunosorbent assay (ELISA), an alternative to the radioimmunoassay for the detection of both antigens and antibodies (27). This technique was later adopted for malaria serology and demonstrated several advantages over the other techniques in use (28). However, in a comparative study with the indirect immunofluorescence and passive hemagglutination tests, it was concluded that the test had the following limitations (29):

a) the persistence of antibodies for prolonged periods made it impossible to distinguish current infection from past infection;

b) the serum antibody titers of persons infected for the first time were generally lower than those of persons who had had malaria on several occasions, which caused false negative results;

c) it was difficult to obtain well-defined antigens from the immunochemical standpoint; and

d) a large number of false negatives occurred in children younger than five years of age.

In any case, the test is specific, is easy to perform, can be automatized, and involves low operating costs. Therefore, it can be used to perform seroepidemiological studies (30, 31). Moreover, it makes it possible to use monoclonal antibodies against specific antigens of each plasmodium species to investigate the presence of antigens, not only in human blood (32) but also in mosquitoes (33, 34).

The application of the immunoenzymatic technique to detect *P. falciparum* antigens in the blood of infected individuals is an important step toward developing a method that will complement microscopic diagnosis (35). Nevertheless, thus far no test has been found that can determine parasitemias lower than those detected through direct microscopic examination or DNA probes (34, 36, 37).

At this point, it has been impossible to reach definitive conclusions on the use of the immunoenzymatic test for diagnostic purposes. In addition to the aforementioned limitations, it will be necessary to solve other problems, such as purification of antigens and test standardization. These problems will be solved because the technique can achieve objective results and allows for an evaluation of the concentration of antibodies after one or two serum dilutions. These properties make it a practical test for establishing the presence not only of immunoglobulins directed against blood forms, but also of specific antibodies directed against other stages of the parasite, as several authors have recently demonstrated (4).

The dot ELISA test is an important variation which is already being used in population surveys of several pathologies (38). It would be helpful to use it in the areas where malaria is endemic, as long as the antigen which is fixed in the solid stage can be standardized. This technique is simple and inexpensive, and it can be done on a large scale.

AGGLUTINATION

Agglutination of infected erythrocytes.   It is possible to make a serologic diagnosis of malaria by using red blood cells from birds with acute infections caused by *P. gallinaceum* (39). Comparison with the indirect immunofluorescence test indicated 99% agreement of the results, but only with the sera of patients with patent parasitemia. The speed with which this test becomes negative suggests that it detects principally IgM antibodies, which could make it an important instrument for epidemiological surveys aimed at determining changes in transmission. Also described was a technique for agglutination of erythrocytes infected by *P. berghei* (40).

The ease with which reagents can be prepared and the prepared product can be standardized, together with the slight technical investment necessary to perform the agglutination tests, encourages more studies in endemic areas to obtain reagents with greater sensitivity and specificity. Thus far, when human red blood cells parasitized by *P. falciparum* have been used as an agglutination reagent for epidemiological purposes, results have not been satisfactory.

Reaction of passive hemagglutination (PH).   Although the initial trials made with this technique using sheep red blood cells sensitized by *P. berghei* as reagent were encouraging, its usefulness was limited by the use of a heterologous antigen (41). The test's problems range from selection of the erythrocytes (humans, sheep, and birds) and their conservation and stabilization (formaldehyde, glutaraldehyde, paraformaldehyde, and pyruvic aldehyde) to the preparation of the antigenic extract for sensitization (42, 43). Several attempts have been made to standardize the PH test, but thus far no reagent is available that would meet the necessary minimum conditions. The work done leads to the conclusion that the technique is not very sensitive in the initial stages of malaria (44). After that period, the test makes it possible to obtain results compatible with those of the IIF. Nevertheless, the lack of uniformity in the preparation of the reagents makes it indispensable to perform more studies. Because it is simple to perform, costs little, and is easy to read—desirable features in the endemic countries—studies should be encouraged to standardize the PH test using well-defined antigens such as peptides obtained through synthesis (antigens of sporozoites or merozoites), in order to make available a test with broad epidemiological application.

PRECIPITATION

Precipitation methods have the advantage of making it possible to differentiate the various systems of antigens and antibodies that appear during the life cycle of the plasmodium in the vertebrate host. It has been observed that in endemic areas the number of precipitant bands increases with age. Since it is less sensitive than other serologic tests, the reaction of precipitation is of little use for diagnosis and it is almost useless for seroepidemiological surveys. Nevertheless, it is useful for identifying the various plasmodial antigenic components, since it makes it possible to differentiate the antigens characteristic of the genus from those of the species.

Soluble *P. falciparum* antigens were identified in the serum of parasitized individuals through double diffusion in agar gel *(45)* and, experimentally, in that of monkeys, birds, and mice *(46)*. The immunoelectrotransference test has also been used to determine the immunochemical profile of individuals infected with different species of plasmodia.

RADIOIMMUNOASSAY

Despite being a third-generation method in its high sensitivity and specificity, radioimmunoassay has been used very little for the immunodiagnosis of malaria. Its use in research on antibodies in serum or on antigens in blood and in mosquitoes yields excellent results both in individual diagnosis and in epidemiological surveys *(32, 47)*. Some of this test's limiting factors in developing countries are its technical complexity, its operative expense, and the short average life of the reagents.

REFERENCES

(1) Vecchio, T. J. Predictive value of a single diagnosis test in unselected populations. *N Engl J Med* 274:1171–1173, 1966.

(2) Deans, J. A., and S. Cohen. Immunology of malaria. *Ann Rev Microbiol* 37:25–49, 1983.

(3) Beaudoin, R. L., J. M. Ramsey, and N. D. Pachedo. Antigens employed in immunodiagnostic tests for the detection of malaria antibodies. WHO/MAL/81.952:1–11. Geneva, 1981.

(4) Moura, R. C. S. Dinâmica da aquisição de imunidade à malária em migrantes da Amazônia (Ariquemes/ RO). Thesis. Faculty of Health Sciences, University of Brasília, 1986.

(5) Wahlgren, M., A. Bjorkman, H. Perlmann, K. Berzins, and P. Perlmann. Anti-*Plasmodium falciparum* antibodies acquired by residents in a holoendemic area of Liberia during development of clinical immunity. *Am J Trop Med Hyg* 35:22–29, 1986.

(6) Voller, A., J. H. E. Th. Meuwissen, and J. P. Verhave. Methods for measuring the immunological response in Plasmodia. Pp. 67–109 *in:* Kreir, J. P. *Malaria.* New York: Academic Press, 1980.

(7) McGregor, I. A. Current concepts concerning man's resistance to infection with malaria. *Bull Soc Pathol Exot* 76:443–445, 1983.

(8) Kagan, I. G. Evaluation of indirect haemagglutination test as an epidemiologic technique for malaria. *Am J Trop Med Hyg* 21:683–689, 1972.

(9) Tobie, J. E., and G. R. Coatney. Fluorescent antibody staining of human malaria parasites. *Exp Parasitol* 11:128–132, 1961.

(10) Kuvin, S. F., J. E. Tobie, C. B. Evans, G. R. Coatney, and P. G. Contacos. Fluorescent antibody studies on the course of antibody production and serum gammaglobulin levels in normal volunteers infected with human and simian malaria. *Am J Trop Med Hyg* 11:429–436, 1962.

(11) Tobie, J. E., S. F. Kuvin, P. G. Contacos, G. R. Coatney, and C. B. Evans. Fluorescent antibody studies on cross reactions between human and simian malaria in normal volunteers. Am J Trop Med Hyg 11:589–596, 1962.

(12) Sulzer, A. J., M. Wilson, and E. C. Hall. Indirect fluorescent-antibody tests for parasitic diseases. V. An evaluation of a thick-smear antigen in the IFA test for malaria antibodies. Am J Trop Med Hyg 18:199–205, 1969.

(13) Ambroise-Thomas, P. L'immunofluorescence dans la serologie du paludisme. WHO/MAL/81.953:1–6. Geneva, 1981.

(14) Sulzer, A. J., A. Turner, and M. Wilson. Preparation of a multi-species antigen of human malaria for use in the indirect fluorescent antibody test. J Parasitol 58:178–179, 1972.

(15) Trager, W., and J. B. Jensen. Human malaria parasites in continuous culture. Science 193:673–675, 1976.

(16) Hall, C. L., J. D. Haynes, J. D. Chulay, and C. L. Diggs. Cultured Plasmodium falciparum used as antigen in a malaria indirect fluorescent antibody test. Am J Trop Med Hyg 27:849–852, 1978.

(17) Ceneviva, A. C. Malária humana: detecção de anticorpos IgM com Plasmodium falciparum de cultura por teste de imunofluorescência. Thesis. Institute of Biomedical Sciences, University of São Paulo, São Paulo, 1983.

(18) World Health Organization. Immunodiagnosis in malaria. WHO/MAL/85.1018:1–18. Geneva, 1985.

(19) Sánchez, M. C. A., V. P. Quartier, S. M. Di Santi, M. Boulos, and A. W. Ferreira. Optimização do teste de imunofluorescência indireta na sorologia da malária humana. Rev Soc Bras Med Trop 20(Suppl):69–70, 1987.

(20) Young, J. F., W. T. Hockmeyer, M. Gross, W. R. Ballou, R. A. Wirtz, J. H. Trosper, R. L. Beaudoin, M. R. Hollingdale, L. H. Miller, C. L. Diggs, and M. Rosenberg. Expression of Plasmodium falciparum circumsporozoite proteins in Escherichia coli for potential use in a human malaria vaccine. Science 228:958–962, 1985.

(21) Howard, R. F., H. A. Stanley, G. H. Campbell, and R. T. Reese. Proteins responsible for a punctate fluorescence pattern in Plasmodium falciparum merozoites. Am J Trop Med Hyg 33:1055–1059, 1984.

(22) Zavala, F., J. P. Tam, M. R. Hollingdale, A. H. Cochrane, I. Quakyi, R. S. Nussenzweig, and V. Nussenzweig. Rationale for development of a synthetic vaccine against Plasmodium falciparum malaria. Science 228:1436–1440, 1985.

(23) Druilhe, P., O. Praderi, J. P. Marc, F. Miltgen, D. Mazier, and G. Parent. Levels of antibodies to Plasmodium falciparum sporozoite surface antigens reflect malaria transmission rates and are persistent in the absence of reinfection. Infect Immun 53:393–397, 1986.

(24) Ram, J. S., P. K. Nakane, D. G. Rawlinson, and G. B. Pierce. Enzyme-labeled antibodies for ultrastructural studies. Fed Proc 25:732–734, 1966.

(25) Nakane, P. K., and G. B. Pierce. Enzyme-labeled antibodies: Preparation and application for the localization of antigens. J Histochem Cytochem 14:929, 1966.

(26) Gentilini, M., and D. Richard-Lenoble. Utilization de marqueurs de la peroxydase pour la recherche et le diagnostic immunologique du paludisme. Bull Soc Path Exot 68:193–197, 1975.

(27) Engvall, E., and P. Perlmann. Enzyme-linked immunosorbent assay (ELISA). Quantitative assay of immunoglobulin G. Immunochemistry 8:871–874, 1971.

(28) Voller, A., D. E. Bidwell, G. Huldt, and E. Engvall. A microplate method of enzyme-linked immunosorbent assay and its application to malaria. Bull WHO 51:209–211, 1974.

(29) Voller, A., R. Cornille-Brogger, J. Storey, and L. Molineaux. A longitudinal study of Plasmodium falciparum malaria in the West African Savana using the ELISA technique. Bull WHO 58:429–438, 1980.

(30) Fandeur, T., and J. P. Dedet. Le test ELISA dans les études séro-épidemiologiques du paludisme humane. Evaluation d'un antigène préparé à partir des hématies de Saimiri sciureus éxperimentalement infectés par Plasmodium falciparum. Bull Soc Pathol Exot 79:50–65, 1986.

(31) Roffin, J., B. Lafabrie, and J. L. Stach. Utilization d'antigènes purifiés pour le sérodiagnostic et les études épidémiologiques du paludisme humain. Intérêt de la technique ELISA pour la mise en évidence des IgG et des IgM spécifiques. Bull Soc Pathol Exot 76:49–68, 1983.

(32) Mackey, L. J., I. A. McGregor, N. Paounova, and P. H. Lambert. Diagnosis of Plasmodium falciparum infection in man: Detection of parasite antigens by ELISA. Bull WHO 60:69–75, 1982.

(33) Arruda, M., M. B. Carvalho, R. S. Nussenzweig, M. Maracic, A. W. Ferreira, and A. H. Cochrane. Potential vectors of malaria and their different susceptibility to Plasmodium falciparum and Plasmodium vivax in Northern Brazil identified by immunoassay. Am J Trop Med Hyg 35:873–881, 1986.

(34) Wirtz, R. A., T. R. Burkot, R. G. André, R. Rosenberg, W. E. Collins, and D. R. Roberts. Identification of Plasmodium vivax sporozoites in mosquitoes using an enzyme-linked immunosorbent assay. Am J Trop Med Hyg 34:1048–1054, 1985.

(35) Mackey, L. J. Tests for the detection of malaria antigens. WHO/MAL/81.957:1–9. Geneva, 1981.

(36) Holmberg, M., A. Bjorkman, L. Franzen, L. Aslund, M. Lebbad, U. Pettersson, and H. Wigzell. Diagnosis of Plasmodium falciparum infection by spot hybridization assay: specificity, sensitivity, and field applicability. Bull WHO 64:579–585, 1986.

(37) World Health Organization. The use of DNA probes for malaria diagnosis. WHO/MAL/86.1022:1–18. Geneva, 1966.

(38) Guimarães, M. C. S., and B. J. Celeste. Soroepidemiologia da leishmaniose mucocutânea: reação de DOT-ELISA em soros da Amazônia e Nordeste do Brasil. *Rev Soc Bras Med Trop* 20(Suppl):135–136, 1987.

(39) Ceneviva, A. C. Reação de aglutinação de hemácias de aves infectadas com *Plasmodium gallinaceum* para pesquisa de anticorpos em málaria humana. Thesis. Faculty of Pharmaceutical Sciences, University of São Paulo, São Paulo, 1975.

(40) Sánchez-Ruiz, M. C. A. Teste de aglutinação de hemácias parasitadas pelo *Plasmodium berghei* na sorologia da malária humana. Thesis. Faculty of Pharmaceutical Sciences, University of São Paulo, São Paulo, 1982.

(41) Desowitz, R. S., and B. Stein. A tanned red cell haemagglutination test using *Plasmodium berghei* and homologous antisera. *Trans R Soc Trop Med Hyg* 56:257–262, 1962.

(42) Kagan, I. G. The indirect haemagglutination and latex tests for malaria serodiagnosis. WHO/MAL/81.954:1–15. Geneva, 1981.

(43) Lunde, M. N., and K. G. Powers. The preparation of malaria haemagglutination antigen. *Ann Trop Med Parasitol* 70:283–291, 1976.

(44) Voller, A., J. H. E. Th. Meuwissen, and T. Goosen. Application of the passive haemagglutination test for malaria: the problem of false negatives. *Bull WHO* 51:662–664, 1974.

(45) Wilson, R. J. M., I. A. McGregor, and M. E. Wilson. The stability and fractionation of malarial antigens from the blood of Africans infected with *Plasmodium falciparum*. *Int J Parasitol* 3:511–520, 1973.

(46) Deans, J. A. Gel diffusion and electrophoretic techniques in the serology of malaria. WHO/MAL/81.956:1–6. Geneva, 1981.

(47) Avraham, H., J. Golenser, D. Bunnag, P. Suntharasamai, S. Tharavanij, K. T. Harinasuta, D. T. Sira, and D. Sulitzeanu. Preliminary field trial of a radioimmunoassay for the diagnosis of malaria. *Am J Trop Med Hyg* 32:11–18, 1983.

Chapter 9

LABORATORY TECHNIQUES

I. SEARCH FOR MALARIA PARASITES IN MOSQUITOES

FILTRATION METHOD

Janine M. Ramsey

MATERIALS AND REAGENTS

1. Mortar
2. Glass wool
3. 10-ml pipettes
4. Syringe with 25-mm and 13-mm Millipore filter unit
5. Whatman #2 filter paper
6. Newbauer hemocytometer
7. Hanks' solution
8. Glutaraldehyde

TEST PROCEDURE

1. Macerate the mosquitoes (up to 100) in a mortar containing a buffer solution (for example, Hanks' buffered saline solution).
2. Filter the macerate, using a 10-ml glass serologic pipette with a 3-cm-long glass wool filter at the tapered end.
3. Run the filtrate through a syringe fixed to a 25-mm Millipore unit containing a premoistened Whatman #2 filter. After this new filtration, collect the suspension in a glass tube.
4. Add glutaraldehyde to the suspension until reaching a final concentration of 1%. Cap the tube and wait at least one hour before proceeding. At this stage the material may be stored for up to six months at 4°C.
5. Centrifuge the samples at 1,500 rpm for 15 minutes.
6. Remove and discard the supernatant. Resuspend the precipitate in 200–400 µl of buffer solution.
7. Filter the resuspended sample through a 13-mm Millipore unit containing a premoistened Whatman #2 filter.
8. Collect the final filtrate and keep it in a capped tube.
9. The sample may be observed immediately or at a later time by phase microscopy. It is recommended that a Newbauer hemocytometer be used to make a quantitative estimate.

Any sample containing two or more sporozoites is considered positive.

TWO-SITE IMMUNOASSAY

Fidel Zavala

MATERIALS AND REAGENTS

1. Plates. Disposable, flexible polyvinyl chloride microtiter plates with a "U" bottom.

2. Monoclonal antibodies. Maintain the purified monoclonal antibodies at a concentration of 1 mg per ml in phosphate-buffered saline solution (PBS). They should be stored at -20 to $-70°C$ in small aliquots (30–100 µl) to avoid repeated freezing and thawing.

3. Labeled antibodies.
   . a) IRMA. Although the ^{125}I labeling can be done with any of the available methods, the Iodogen technique is preferred.
   b) ELISA. Labeling with peroxidase gives good results, and the preferred technique is the one described by Nakane and Kawaoi.[1]

4. Enzyme substrates. Two different substrates have been used: OPD (O-phenylene diamine) and ABTS (2,2'-azino-di-(3-ethylbenzthiazoline)-6-sulfonic acid). OPD: Dissolve in methanol to a concentration of 10 mg per ml. Then dilute 100 times in distilled water and add hydrogen peroxide to a final concentration of 0.003%. ABTS: Dissolve 1 mg per ml in a 0.1 M citrate buffer solution, pH 4.0. Add hydrogen peroxide to a final concentration of 0.003%. The substrate solution should be prepared immediately before use.

5. Buffer solutions.
   a) Blocking buffer (BB). A phosphate-buffered saline solution (PBS) containing 1% bovine serum albumin, 0.5% casein, and 0.01% thimerosal.
   b) Washing buffer (WB). PBS containing 0.05% Tween 20.
   c) Grinding buffer (GB). Blocking buffer solution containing 0.5% Nonidet P-40 (NP-40) as detergent.

6. Mosquito extract. With a sealed Pasteur pipette, triturate the mosquito in 30 µl of GB. The trituration may be done in plastic tubes or in hard microtiter plates with U-shaped wells. If the extract is not used immediately, store at -20 to $-70°C$. Before performing the assay, add 130–200 µl of BB to each sample.

ASSAY PROCEDURE

The first four steps apply to both the IRMA and ELISA techniques.

1. Incubate the wells of the plastic plate with 30 µl of monoclonal antibody diluted in PBS to a final concentration of 10 micrograms (µg) per ml.

2. After overnight incubation at room temperature, wash the wells three times with BB. Fill the wells again with BB and incubate 30–60 minutes at room temperature.

---

[1]Peroxidase-labeled antibody: A new method of conjugation. *J Histochem Cytochem* 22:1084–1091, 1974.

3. Discard the BB in the wells through aspiration and add 30 μl of mosquito extract. Incubate for two hours at room temperature.

4. Wash the wells three times with WB, and add 30 μl of labeled antibody.

IRMA

5. Add 30 μl of ^{125}I-labeled antibody (100,000 counts per minute) diluted in BB.

6. Incubate for one hour at room temperature. Wash thoroughly with WB, dry, and place individually in a gamma counter.

ELISA

5. Add 30 μl of antibody labeled with peroxidase to a concentration of 1 μg per ml diluted in BB.

6. Incubate for one hour at room temperature and then wash three times with WB.

7. Add 50 μl of substrate solution and incubate for 30–60 minutes in darkness.

8. If OPD is used, stop the reaction with 8N sulfuric acid and read the absorbance at 494 nm. If ABTS is used, stop the reaction with 1 M sodium fluoride and read the absorbance at 414 nm.

II. MICROSCOPIC DIAGNOSIS IN BLOOD[1]

Francisco J. López-Antuñano

PREPARATION OF THICK FILM

A thick blood film should show the blood elements uniformly distributed on the microscope slide. This type of preparation makes it possible not only to obtain an idea of the number of parasites in the blood, but also to make a quick and efficient diagnosis of the malarial species. Since the cells are concentrated, it is the best way to quickly find limited parasitemias.

A thick film must not be too thick[2] and it should be centered in the middle third of the slide, leaving a space of at least 1.5 cm at each end to allow for handling during the staining process.

---

[1]Revised version of Parts II.7 and II.9 through II.11 of the *Manual for the Microscopic Diagnosis of Malaria*, 4th edition. Scientific Publication No. 276. Washington, D.C., Pan American Health Organization, 1975.

[2]To determine whether a sample is too thick, the slide is set up on its edge while the blood is moist. If the blood runs toward the slide's supporting edge, it must be spread until it no longer runs, but rather hardly moves.

Normal practice is to place one single sample on each slide. However, when many samples are being taken in large-scale surveys or when the personnel evaluating the specimens must carry considerable amounts of material and equipment during long field visits, up to five samples may be placed on the same slide, as long as a free space of at least 1.5 cm is always left at each end.

Sterile disposable needles or lancets should be used for puncturing the skin. The puncture site is cleansed of dirt and sweat with 95% alcohol and gauze. Long-fiber cotton may also be used.

The following steps are to be followed in preparing a thick film (Figure 9.1):

1. All necessary data concerning the patient and the person collecting the sample must be properly recorded in order to prevent any error in the patient's identification.

2. Two slides are used, and it is essential that they be meticulously clean. They should be held by the edges at the ends, between the thumb and index finger, to avoid any contact with the surfaces.

3. The skin to be punctured is firmly wiped with a piece of alcohol-moistened gauze, and then dried with another piece of clean gauze. Blood may be taken from the index finger, from the ear lobe if it is fleshy enough, or, in the case of small children, from the big toe or heel. If the index finger is chosen, the side rather than the tip should be punctured.

4. The cover of the sterile disposable lancet or needle is removed.

5. The individual collecting the blood firmly holds the finger to be punctured between his or her thumb and index finger. The puncture is made with a quick jab of the lancet or needle held in the other hand.

6. The first drop of blood is cleaned away with dry gauze.

7. The finger is squeezed gently to obtain another drop of blood, taking care not to press the puncture point. A spherical drop of blood is allowed to well up on the dry skin.

8. The clean slide is held by the edges at one end, and an edge at the other end is pressed for support against the collector's index finger (which is squeezing the donor's finger). The slide is eased down until it makes contact with the drop of blood. If the amount of blood is insufficient, a second drop may be placed close to the first one. The donor's finger must not be allowed to touch the slide.

9. The slide is placed face up on the work surface. Using the corner and the first 5 mm of the long edge of the second slide, the collector spreads the blood to form a square or rectangle of the appropriate size and thickness. The slide used to spread the blood is cleaned immediately to avoid transferences from one sample to another. If more than one sample from the same donor is needed, the next drop is picked up with the clean corner of the spreader slide, is placed close to the first sample, and is spread directly with that slide.

10. After the donor's finger has been wiped off, a smaller drop of the excess blood is collected with the corner of the spreader slide.

11. This blood is placed on the slide some 5 mm below the already-spread drop or drops, leaving enough space to write the necessary identification.

12. Once the necessary amount of blood has been obtained, the donor's finger is cleaned with alcohol-moistened gauze.

13. The sample is placed on the work surface and is fanned briskly with a piece of cardboard to dry it.

14. When the sample is dry, the collector's identification, the sample's serial number, and the date on which the blood was taken are noted in the area of the slide kept blank for that purpose.

15. In the event several specimens are required, five narrow thick films are placed across the same slide. Accordingly, less blood is taken per sample and the samples are spread over a smaller area. The same spreader slide is used in all the operations. The first drop is placed to the left for identification purposes, and as soon as the blood dries, the serial number is noted in the proper place.

Always placing the sample in the same portion of the slide saves much time in locating the blood under the microscope. Figure 9.2 shows a guide with the appropriate dimensions for this purpose. Obviously, when a single slide is used for several samples, a different guide must be followed.

STAINING TECHNIQUES

A thick blood film on a nearly rectangular 1.5-by-1.2 cm area can contain 6 to 20 times the amount of blood in a thin smear. Whereas it is relatively easy to see through a single layer of stained red blood cells, when thick film red cells are "fixed" nothing can be seen except perhaps at the edges of the preparation. It is therefore necessary to remove the hemoglobin from the erythrocytes, either before or during the staining process. In the past, distilled water, weak hydrochloric acid solutions, or other mixtures were used to remove the hemoglobin before the stain was added. This often caused not only lysis and complete destruction of the red blood cells, but also lysis and deformation of the parasites, the leukocytes, and other blood elements. Later, a method was developed of dehemoglobinization with the staining solution.

Time, alcohol, and heat "fix" the hemoglobin in red blood cells. Therefore, the more promptly thick films can be stained, the more complete the dehemoglobinization will be. Conversely, the longer they remain unstained, the less clear the preparations will be. A thick film remaining unstained for 7 to 10 days in a warm and humid climate may not be suitable for examination.

Originally, thick film samples were stained by covering a rather large thick drop of blood with diluted methylene blue. Since visibility in the central portion was virtually nil, it was thought that examination would be easier if the blood were thoroughly stirred. Then followed a long period in which defibrination was considered imperative, until it was realized that merely a little less blood in the drop gave the desired results. The stain that used to be used almost exclusively was one drop of Giemsa per 1 ml distilled water. The diluted Giemsa stain was added to the thick film and allowed to act for approximately an hour, after which the slides were dried and examined.

Following the discovery of the dehemoglobinizing action of isotonic solutions of methylene blue, a quick staining method for thick films was developed. It consisted of submersing the samples for one to three seconds in solution A (a mixture of methylene blue, azure A, and phosphates), followed by briefly washing them in distilled water and then dipping them for the same length of time in solution B (a mixture of eosin and phosphates). Although the method succeeded in highlighting both the leukocytes and the parasites in clear, bright colors, it was too fast to allow for complete dehemoglobinization.

When samples can be stained at the laboratory within a week, the complete process can be carried out without really affecting dehemoglobinization or the results of staining. Nevertheless, when more than a week's delay is expected, the first step of Walker's method (see below) should be done in the field within a few days after blood collection in order to avoid "fixation."

If six weeks or more elapse before staining is begun, especially in the tropics, the blood samples may be completely ruined, since proper dehemoglobinization and staining will not be possible. Thus far all methods of dehemoglobinization and staining of overdried or "fixed" thick films have failed. Although poorly stained blood samples can be stained again in various ways and sometimes with satisfactory results, there is no known technique capable of restoring blood smears that have been allowed to become too dry.

WALKER'S METHOD (FIGURES 9.3 AND 9.4)

First Step

1. Dip the slide for one second in a solution of methylene blue. Briefly touch the slide's free end to a moistened plastic sponge or small pad in order to remove the excess blue and thus reduce the number of times the buffer solution must be changed.

2. Rinse with a buffer solution until the margins of the thick film become a light bluish gray. Do not proceed to the wash until the red color leaves every part of the drop. Five gentle dips in buffer solution are sufficient. If dealing with more than ten slides, use two wide-mouthed glasses and change the buffer solution when it becomes too blue.

3. Allow the slides to drain in a rack. When Giemsa stain cannot be used immediately after completing the above procedure:

- Dry the slides with gentle heat or in sunlight to avoid fungus growth.
- Wrap the slides in packets of 5 to 15 and store them in a dry place until they can be stained with Giemsa solution (see below).

Second Step

4. Place the inverted slides over the 2–3 mm well of the staining plate or on an enameled tray.

5. Allow a recently prepared aqueous solution of Giemsa stain (one drop Giemsa alcoholic solution to 1 ml buffer solution) to run under the slide until the well is filled. Eliminate any bubbles that may form under or near the thick blood film.

6. Allow the stain to act for 6 to 10 minutes. Staining time may vary from one lot of stain to another and it should be carefully monitored for best results.

7. Briefly dip the slides twice in buffer solution to remove excess Giemsa stain.

8. Drain, then dry with gentle heat and fanning.

9. Examine with oil-immersion objective.

FIELD'S METHOD

1. Dip in solution A for one to three seconds.
2. Wash gently in buffer solution.
3. Dip in solution B for one to four seconds.
4. Wash gently in buffer solution.
5. Drain, then dry with gentle heat and fanning.

The rapidity of this method does not allow complete dehemoglobinization of the thick film as does the methylene blue-Giemsa technique. However, the border colors are almost the same with both methods, and they last longer with this technique.

ROMANOWSKY'S METHOD (MODIFIED) (FIGURE 9.5)

1. Place the inverted slides over the 2–3 mm well in the plastic staining plate.
2. Allow a recently prepared mixture of diluted solution A and double-strength solution B to run under the slide until the well is filled. Eliminate any bubbles that may form under or near the thick film. To dilute solution A, use 5 ml of buffer for each one or two drops of double-strength solution. To dilute the final mixture, use 5 ml of diluted solution A for each drop of double-strength solution B.
3. Let the stain act for 10 minutes.
4. Briefly dip the slide in buffer solution to remove the excess stain.
5. Drain, then dry with gentle heat and fanning.
6. Examine with oil-immersion objective.

REMARKS

Similar results have been obtained using a diluted mixture of azure-methylene blue-eosin instead of aqueous Giemsa stain, applied after the thick film has been treated with methylene blue phosphate (Walker's method, first step). It is important that the stain be prepared immediately before use, since the methylene blue-eosin precipitates out after the aqueous solutions are mixed.

FORMULAS FOR PREPARATION OF STAINS

WALKER'S METHOD

Methylene blue phosphate

Methylene blue chloride (medicinal)	1.0 g
Sodium phosphate, anhydrous (Na_2HPO_4)	3.0 g
Potassium phosphate (KH_2PO_4)	1.0 g

Mix thoroughly in a dry mortar. One gram of the mixture is dissolved into 250–350 ml of distilled water and filtered if necessary.

Alcohol solution of Giemsa stain

Giemsa stain powder, certified[3]	0.75 g
Pure methyl alcohol (acetone-free)	65.0 ml
Pure glycerin	35.0 ml

Shake well 6 to 10 times a day in a bottle containing glass beads until it is well mixed. Always keep tightly closed and filter when it breaks up.

FIELD'S METHOD

Solution A

Methylene blue chloride (medicinal)	0.8 g
Azure I or azure B (certified)	0.5 g

Dissolve in 500 ml of buffer solution.

Solution B

Eosin Yellow, water soluble	1.0 g

Dissolve in 500 ml of buffer solution.

To keep the solutions free of contamination and precipitates, they should be kept in plastic dropper bottles, from which they can be poured over dry thick films for quick staining.

ROMANOWSKY'S METHOD (MODIFIED)

Solution A (double strength)

Methylene blue chloride (medicinal)	0.8 g
Azure I or azure B	0.5 g

Dissolve in 250 ml of buffer solution.

Solution B (double strength)

Eosin Yellow, water soluble	1.0 g

Dissolve in 250 ml of buffer solution.

For in-the-field staining, solution A prediluted in the recommended proportion (one or two drops per 5 ml buffer solution) may be used. Immediately before staining, one drop of solution B is added for each 5 ml of diluted solution A.

---

[3]If Giemsa powder is not available, Wright's powder may be used in the same proportion.

BUFFER SOLUTION

Sodium phosphate, anhydrous[4] (Na_2HPO_4)	4 g
Potassium phosphate (KH_2PO_4)	5 g

Mix well in a mortar and dissolve 1 g of the mixture in one liter of distilled water.

REMARKS

The amounts of stain powder and salts indicated above are only averages, and may be varied according to the results obtained. For example, if a Giemsa powder gives especially good results when dissolved in a certain proportion with glycerin and alcohol, then that proportion should be used. An attempt should likewise be made to find the mixture of salts for the buffer solution that will give the best results. Sodium phosphate (SP) and potassium phosphate (PP) crystals are weighed in proportions of 1:5, 2:5, 4:5, 6:5, 8:5, and 10:5. Several preparations of the same blood should be stained with the same Giemsa using different buffer solutions prepared by adding 1 g of the salt mixture to a liter of distilled water. The buffer solution giving the best results is then used. The proportion of 4:5 is the one most often chosen. The pH of these mixtures varies from 6.26 to 7.20.[5]

If the alcohol solution is too strong and the cellular components are overstained, five or six drops in 10 ml of diluent will be enough to correct the problem. Nevertheless, it is more desirable to dilute the stain with more of the alcohol-glycerin mixture in order to maintain the universal proportion of one drop of alcoholic stain solution to 1 ml of buffer solution.

Staining times may also vary from one stain lot to another and therefore should be tested meticulously.

EVALUATION OF THE PREPARATION AND STAINING
OF THICK BLOOD FILMS

Examination of thick films should begin by systematically analyzing the blood elements and parasites (Figure 9.6) for the shapes and colors obtained and by verifying that there has been sufficient dehemoglobinization of the red blood cells. The absence of platelets indicates an unusual condition in the blood itself or the addition of a foreign substance. An abundance of distorted leukocytes with abnormally shaped nuclei indicates that the diluent was unsuitable. If the red cells appear to be "fixed" and stain as a thick dark background, dehemoglobinization was not adequate. Under such circumstances the specimen cannot be properly examined.

The best staining is obtained when the thick film is spread uniformly, dried quickly, and treated with high-quality stains and diluents. A well-prepared and properly stained sample should have the following features:

---

[4]*Primary sodium phosphate*: 1.25 g of Na_2HPO_4 + $2H_2O$ = 1 g of anhydrous Na_2HPO_4. *Sodium phosphate crystals*: 12.6 g of Na_2HPO_4 + $12H_2O$ = 5 g of anhydrous Na_2HPO_4; 2.5 g of Na_2HPO_4 + $12H_2O$ = 1 g of anhydrous Na_2HPO_4.

[5]pH: 6.26, 6.50, 6.90, 7.05, 7.10, and 7.20 for salt proportions (SP/PP) 1:5, 2:5, 4:5, 6:5, 8:5, and 10:5, respectively.

Dehemoglobinization.   The background of the sample must be transparent and as light as possible.

Thickness.   There should be an average of 10 to 20 leukocytes per microscopic field (oil immersion).

Colors.   The colors of the elements should be checked routinely and in the same order, as follows:

Red cell remains: blue
Platelets: deep pink to violet
Nuclei of leukocytes: generally deep blue to violet
Leukocyte granules:
  Neutrophils: some pink, some blue, and some violet in the same cell
  Eosinophils: dark copperish red
Cytoplasm of the lymphocytes: pale blue
Cytoplasm of the monocytes: blue

If the blood elements do not have those colors, it is unlikely that the parasites' chromatin or cytoplasm is stained to the appropriate color. However, a sample with well-stained parasites may contain poorly stained blood components, and vice versa. Old or destroyed blood elements and parasites usually stain poorly.

III. DETECTION OF ANTIBODIES

Antonio Walter Ferreira

INDIRECT IMMUNOFLUORESCENCE TECHNIQUE[1]

REAGENTS

Antigens

Plasmodium falciparum and *P. vivax* obtained from the blood of individuals with a recent primary infection or from continuous *in vitro* culture.

Sera

1. Positive control sera with known antibody titer.
2. Negative control sera.
3. Reference sera.
4. Sera for testing.

[1]Source: López-Antuñano, F. J. Standardization of Indirect Immunoflourescence (IIF) Tests for Malaria. PAHO/WHO, Internal Memorandum, 1984, 15 pages.

Fluorescent conjugates

Anti-IgG sheep or goat immunoglobulins and anti-IgM human immunoglobulins specific for γ and μ chains, labeled with fluorescein isothiocyanate to obtain an F/P molar ratio between 3.5 and 4.5.

Buffer solutions

1. Phosphate-buffered saline solution (PBS), 0.01 M, pH 7.2

NaCl	8.183 g
Na_2HPO_4	1.051 g
NaH_2PO_4	0.310 g
Distilled H_2O, to final volume of	1,000 ml

2. PBS solution with 1% Tween 80

Tween 80	1 ml
PBS 0.01 M, pH 7.2	99 ml

3. Carbonate/bicarbonate buffer solution, 0.5 M, pH 8.5

   Solution A

Na_2CO_3	5.3 g
Distilled H_2O, to final volume of	100 ml

   Solution B

$NaHCO_3$	4.2 g
Distilled H_2O, to final volume of	100 ml

Mix 0.4 ml of solution A and 10 ml of solution B. Confirm that the pH is 8.5. If it is not, add solution A or B until the desired pH is reached.

4. Buffered glycerin for the slide assembly.

Mix nine parts of twice-distilled glycerin and one part of the carbonate/bicarbonate buffer solution, 0.5 M, pH 8.5.

5. Evans blue solution

   Concentrated solution

Evans blue	10 mg
PBS-Tween 80, to final volume of	100 ml

   Solution for use
   Dilute to 1/5 concentrated solution at the time of use, as follows:

Concentrated solution	2 parts
PBS-Tween 80	8 parts

Solution for staining parasites (Giemsa stain)

1. Stain solution

Giemsa stain powder	0.75 g
Methyl alcohol	65.0 ml
Glycerin	35.0 ml

Shake 6 to 10 times per day in an amber-colored flask containing glass beads until it is well mixed. Keep tightly closed at all times. Filter when removed from flask for use.

2. Buffer solution

Na_2HPO_4	4 g
KH_2PO_4	5 g

Mix well and dissolve 1 g of the mixture in 1 liter of distilled water.

Solution for ripening parasites

PBS-glucose

Glucose U.S.P.	0.5 g
PBS[2]	100 ml

After adding the glucose, filter through a 0.22-micron Millipore filter.

PREPARATION OF ANTIGENS

Obtaining *P. falciparum* and *P. vivax* antigens from parasitized human blood

1. Collect the blood with anticoagulant.
2. Prepare a complete blood smear and stain it following Giemsa's method to count the number of parasitized red blood cells per microscopic field (See Chapter 9.II). Good antigens are obtained when the blood used has a minimum parasitemia of 1.0% and schizonts predominate.

3a. Preparation of *Plasmodium falciparum* antigens: As soon as the blood with anticoagulant is collected, it is incubated for 24 hours at 37°C after diluting it by one half with PBS-glucose. Then, centrifuge the blood at 2,500 rpm for five minutes, and discard the supernatant and layer of leukocytes.

3b. Preparation of *Plasmodium vivax* antigens: As soon as the blood is collected, it should be centrifuged at 2,500 rpm for five minutes. Discard the plasma and the layer of leukocytes. This operation should be done carefully because the parasitized red blood cells are immediately below the layer of leukocytes.

4. Wash the red cells four times by centrifuging at 2,500 rpm for five minutes in a volume of PBS 10 times greater than the volume of the erythrocyte sediment.

5. Resuspend the washed sediment in a suitable volume of PBS, which depends on the number of plasmodia per microscopic field. The dilution factor can be figured with the following formula: $VD = (2.5 \times N) - 1$, where VD is the volume of diluent in parts that should be added to one part of the sediment volume, and N is the number of schizont-parasitized red blood cells per microscopic field.

6. Deposit 5 µl of the suspension obtained onto a delimited area of the slide.
7. Dry the slides at room temperature.
8. Store the slides at −70°C in a humidity-free environment after wrapping them first individually in absorbent paper and then in groups of 10 in aluminum foil or in a sealed plastic bag.

---

[2]Previously sterilized in an autoclave for 20 minutes at 120°C at one atmosphere of pressure.

Obtaining *P. falciparum* antigen from *in vitro* culture

Good results are obtained with synchronized cultures with a high density of schizonts in RPMI 1640 media. The same procedure is used as for the preparation of *P. vivax* antigen from parasitized human blood.

EVALUATION OF THE ANTIGENS PREPARED

The quality of each new batch of antigens should be evaluated by using the following controls:

1. Positive standard sera of known titer.
2. Negative standard sera.
3. Reference serum.
4. Reagents used in the test.

TITRATION OF THE CONJUGATE

It is necessary to assay the activity of each new batch of conjugate used with the different batches of antigen. This is done by block titration, using a battery of known positive and negative standard sera. The titer of the conjugate is considered to be the largest dilution that provides maximum sensitivity and specificity.

EXECUTION OF THE TEST

1. When they are to be used, take the slides out of the freezer and place them in a desiccator containing silica gel until they reach room temperature.
2. Double the dilution of the sera in PBS-Tween 80 starting from a 1:8 dilution.
3. Cover the areas on the slides containing the antigen with 20 μl of the serum dilution.
4. Incubate the slides at 37°C for 30 minutes in a moist chamber.
5. Wash the plates twice in PBS and then leave them in that solution for 10 minutes.
6. Drain off the excess PBS and dry the edges of the specimen areas with filter paper.
7. Place over each area containing antigen 20 μl of conjugate diluted according to the titer in a solution of PBS-Tween 80 that contains Evans blue at a concentration of 2 mg per 100 ml.
8. Incubate for 30 minutes at 37°C in a moist chamber and wash the slides as directed in paragraph 5.
9. Rinse, dry, and mount the slides using buffered glycerin and a coverslip.
10. Observe the preparations with a fluorescent microscope (40× immersion objective and 10× eyepiece).

Whatever the number of samples prepared, the following controls must be used:

a) Antigen + PBS + conjugate.
b) Antigen + negative standard serum + conjugate.
c) Antigen + positive standard serum + conjugate.
d) Unparasitized red blood cells + positive standard serum + conjugate.

e) Unparasitized red blood cells + negative standard serum + conjugate.

f) Unparasitized red blood cells + serum to be tested + conjugate.

The fluorescent reaction should be observed only in the positive control serum in the presence of the antigen.

INTERPRETATION OF THE TEST

1. The highest dilution that shows well-defined fluorescence over the parasite's entire surface will be considered the serum's titer. Plasmodia do not show fluorescence in negative reactions.

2. The threshold of reactivity for IgG antibodies is normally a dilution of 1:16, and that for IgM antibodies, 1:32.

CAUSES OF ERROR

False positives

1. Presence of the rheumatoid factor. IgG and IgM antibody sera should be tested for the presence of this factor (latex test). If positive, the rheumatoid factor should be absorbed with immunoglobulin polymerized by glutaraldehyde or similarly acting commercial products and the sera should be assayed again for the presence of specific IgM antibodies.

2. Poorly titrated conjugates.

3. Cross-reactions between different species of plasmodia.

4. Presence of autoantibodies.

5. Mixture of different sera on the slides due to confluence.

False negatives

1. Inadequate storage of the reagents.

2. Insufficient illumination of the microscope.

3. Poorly titrated conjugates.

4. Control sera lacking immunologic activity.

5. Sera with antibodies directed against restricted epitopes of the parasite.

REMARKS

An interesting alternative way of carrying out the IIF test is to collect blood on filter paper from the fingertip or earlobe.[3] The sample may then be stored for several months at 4°C in a dry place and later processed, with serum for the test being obtained by submerging the filter paper in PBS.[3,4] Experiments show that the IgM antibodies lose their activity more rapidly than the IgG antibodies.[4]

---

[3]Srinivasa, H., and P. Bhat. Evaluation of micro-sampling of blood by filter paper strips for malaria seroepidemiology. *Indian J Malariol* 21:127–129, 1984.

[4]Guimaraes, M. C. S., E. A. Castilho, B. J. Celeste, O. S. Nakahara, and V. Amato Neto. Almacenamiento a largo plazo de IgG e IgM en papel filtro para su uso en encuestas seroepidemiológicas de enfermedades parasitarias. *Bol Of Sanit Panam* 100:129–142, 1986.

ENZYME-LINKED IMMUNOSORBENT ASSAY TECHNIQUE (ELISA)[5]

REAGENTS

Antigens

Soluble antigenic components of *P. falciparum* or *P. vivax* obtained from persons with recent primary infection or from a continuous *in vitro* culture.

Sera

1. Positive control sera.
2. Negative control sera.
3. Reference sera.
4. Sera for testing.

Conjugates

Anti-IgG sheep or goat immunoglobulins and anti-IgM human immunoglobulins labeled with peroxidase.

Buffer solutions

1. Phosphate-buffered saline solution (PBS), 0.01 M, pH 7.2, containing 0.05% Tween 20

NaCl	8.183 g
Na_2HPO_4	1.051 g
NaH_2PO_4	0.310 g
Distilled H_2O, to final volume of	1,000 ml

Add 0.5 ml of Tween 20 to 1,000 ml of PBS.

2. Carbonate-bicarbonate buffer solution, 0.06 M, pH 9.6

Solution A

Sodium carbonate	3.18 g
Distilled H_2O, to final volume of	500 ml

Solution B

Sodium bicarbonate	2.52 g
Distilled H_2O, to final volume of	500 ml

While shaking constantly, add enough solution B to solution A to obtain the desired pH.

---

[5]Ambroise-Thomas, P., J. Thelu, and F. Peyron. *Plasmodium falciparum* antibodies. *In*: Bergmeyer, H. U. *Methods of Enzymatic Analysis*. Weinhein, VCH Verlaggesellschaft 11:311–325, 1986.

3. Phosphate-citric acid buffer solution
    Solution A
    Na_2HPO_4 11.9 g
    Distilled H_2O, to final volume of   1,000 ml

    Solution B
    Citric acid   7.0 g
    Distilled H_2O, to final volume of   1,000 ml

Mix enough solution A with solution B, while shaking constantly, to obtain a pH of 4.9 to 5.2.

4. Buffer solution of carbonate-bicarbonate and bovine serum albumin (BSA)
    BSA (fraction V)   1.0 g
    Buffer solution of carbonate-bicarbonate,
        0.06 M, pH 9.6, to final volume of   100 ml

5. Chromogen solution
    OPD (orthophenylene diamine-HCl)   10 mg
    Phosphate-citric acid buffer solution, pH 5.0   25 ml
    H_2O_2, 30%   10 µl

6. HCl 1N

7. Extraction buffer solution
    Urea   48.0 g
    PBS, to final volume of   100 ml

Culture Medium

Basic RPMI 1640 culture medium

1. Dissolve 10.4 g of RPMI 1640 in 900 ml bidistilled water. Add 5.94 g of Hepes and bring to a final volume of 960 ml.
2. Pass through a 0.22 µm Millipore filter.
3. Add 100 µg of neomycin.

Buffered RPMI medium

1. Before using, add 4.2 ml of 5% $NaHCO_3$ for each 100 ml of the basic medium.
2. Measure the pH and, if necessary, adjust to pH 7.2 with NaOH 1 M or HCl 1 M.

RPMI medium with 0.04% saponin

    Saponin   0.04 g
    Buffered RPMI medium, to final volume of   100 ml

Enrichment of the suspensions of parasitized red blood cells

1. Centrifuge the parasitized red blood cells taken from culture at 2,500 rpm for 10 minutes.
2. Wash the sediment twice with a volume of the buffered culture medium five times greater than that of the sediment.
3. Centrifuge at 1,500 rpm for 10 minutes.
4. Prepare a 20% suspension of red blood cells in buffered culture medium.
5. Add an equal volume of plasmagel.
6. Shake constantly until the sample is homogenized.
7. Incubate in a water bath at 37°C for 30 minutes.
8. Remove the upper layer containing the red blood cells parasitized with schizonts.
9. Centrifuge at 2,000 rpm for 10 minutes.
10. Discard the supernatant and suspend the sediment with an equal volume of buffered culture medium.
11. Determine the parasitemia in the suspension by means of Giemsa staining. Antigen can be obtained from suspensions with a level of parasitized red blood cells of 40% or higher.
12. Wash the parasitized red cells twice with a volume of buffered culture medium five times greater than that of the sediment.

Lysis of the prepared erythrocytes

1. Add to the enriched sediment of parasitized red blood cells a solution of 0.04% saponin in buffered culture medium.
2. Shake the sample rapidly to homogenize it and incubate at room temperature for 20 minutes.
3. Centrifuge at 3,000 rpm for 15 minutes and wash the sediment twice with the buffered culture medium.

Extraction of the plasmodium antigens

1. Suspend the sediment obtained above in the extraction buffer solution.
2. Sonicate at 30 hertz for 30 seconds at 30-second intervals for four minutes.
3. Centrifuge at 12,000 rpm at 4°C for 30 minutes.
4. Discard the sediment, remove the supernatant, and freeze in liquid nitrogen at $-70°C$.

Determination of the protein concentration of the supernatant

This is done using the Warbung-Christian spectrophotometric method.

Use polystyrene plates with 96 wells. Place in each well 50 μl of antigen diluted in carbonate-bicarbonate buffer solution, 0.06 M, pH 9.6. The antigen's proper dilution for use is determined by block titration. The plates with the antigen are incubated at 37°C for two hours and then kept at 4°C for 18 hours.

EXECUTION OF THE TEST (ELISA)

1. Remove the plates from the refrigerator and wash three times with PBS-Tween 20 0.05% for five minutes.
2. Add to each plate well 200 μl of a 1% solution of BSA in carbonate-bicarbonate buffer solution (0.06 M, pH 9.6), and incubate at 37°C for one hour to block any unspecific reaction.
3. Wash the plates three times with PBS-Tween 20 0.05% for five minutes.
4. Add 50 μl of each serum dilution to the plate's wells. The control and reference sera should be titrated and the test sera should be diluted to 1/50 and 1/100. All the sera should be diluted in PBS with 0.05% Tween 20.
5. Incubate at 37°C for two hours in a humid chamber.
6. Wash the plates as indicated in paragraph 3.
7. Add 50 μl of the enzyme-labeled conjugate, diluted according to its titer in PBS with 0.05% Tween 20, to each well and incubate at 37°C for one hour.
8. Wash the plates as indicated in paragraph 3.
9. Add 100 μl of recently prepared chromogen solution, homogenize, and incubate for 15 minutes away from light.
10. Block the enzymatic reaction with 50 μl of 1N HCl.
11. Read by sight or by spectrophotometry at 492 nm.

CALCULATION OF THE SERUM TITER

The titer of the sera can be calculated based on one or two dilutions, until there is a linear relationship between the dilution and the optical density.[6]

1. The following formula is used for one dilution of the serum:

$$T = \log D + \frac{\log OD - \log OD \text{ "cut off"}}{K}$$

$$K = \frac{\delta \log OD}{\delta \log D}$$

where D = dilution of the serum; OD = optical density of dilution D at 492 nm; OD "cut off" = optical density at 492 nm of the reactivity threshold between reactive and nonreactive sera; and K = relationship between the variation in OD and the variation in the dilutions of control sera, given by the slope of a graphed straight line.

2. The following formula is used for two dilutions of sera:

$$T = \log D_1 + \frac{(\log OD_1 - \log OD \text{ "cut off"}) \times (\log D_2 - \log D_1)}{\log OD_1 - \log OD_2}$$

[6]Camargo, M. E., L. Silveira, J. A. Furuta, E. P. T. Oliveira, and O. A. Germek. Immunoenzymatic assay of anti-diphtheric toxin antibodies in human serum. *J Clin Microbiol* 20:772–774, 1984.

where D_1 and D_2 = dilutions of serum, and OD_1 and OD_2 = optical densities of dilutions D_1 and D_2, respectively.

3. Determination of the "cut off." The "cut off" is determined with 15 to 20 nonreactive sera using the formula "cut off" = $\overline{X}$ + 2 SD, where $\overline{X}$ = arithmetic mean of the optical densities of the nonreactive sera and SD = standard deviation.

INTERPRETATION OF THE TEST

1. The results of the ELISA test can be expressed in titers or in absorbance. In the latter case, a blank should give a reading below 0.100 and negative sera should give readings up to 0.200. The sera are considered positive when the corrected readings are above 0.500.

2. A mixture of all of the test's reagents, with the exception of the serum sample, should be used as the blank for calibrating the spectrophotometer at zero.

CAUSES OF ERROR

False positives

1. Cross-reactions between different plasmodia.
2. Poorly blocked plates.
3. Poorly titrated antigens and conjugates.
4. Altered chromogen solution.
5. Rheumatoid factor.
6. Unsuitable plastic plates.

False negatives

1. Poorly titrated antigens and conjugates.
2. Excess blocker.
3. Altered chromogen solution.
4. Unsuitable plastic plates.

REMARKS

1. The optimal amounts and concentrations of the various reagents depend on their individual characteristics.

2. The serum samples may be diluted 1:50 and 1:100 with the appropriate buffer solutions to determine the titer.

3. The optimal concentrations of the antigens and conjugates should be determined by block titration.

4. The serum samples should be examined in duplicate or triplicate.

5. In each plastic plate, positive and negative control sera, diluted in series, should be tested so that the titers of the samples under study can be determined in one or two dilutions, according to the daily conditions of the reaction.

6. The amounts of the components used in the ELISA may vary in accordance with the standardization established by each laboratory.

7. The incubation periods of the various stages of the ELISA technique may be adjusted according to local conditions.

8. The sera and conjugate are to be diluted with a buffer solution containing 1% BSA.

9. The literature contains innumerable variations with regard to preparation of the antigen, some of which indicate that it is possible to extract the antigenic components without concentrating the schizonts with plasmagel. To remove the remains of the red blood cell membranes, the antigen can be centrifuged in a Ficoll gradient P 400 at 27% (P/V). The antigen can also be sonicated in PBS.

FIGURES

CREDITS

Fig. 1.1: Photograph provided by Dr. Manuel Martínez Báez.

Fig. 2.1, 2.2, 2.3, 2.4: Photographs provided by Dr. Abdu Azad, University of Maryland, Baltimore, MD, USA.

Fig. 3.1, 3.3, 3.4, 3.5: Photographs provided by Dr. R. W. Gwadz.

Fig. 3.2: Reproduced with the permission of the publisher from M. Katz, D. D. Despommier, and R. W. Gwadz. Life Cycle. In: *Parasitic Diseases*, New York, Springer-Verlag, Inc., 1982.

Fig. 4.1: Reprinted with modifications from *Terminology of Malaria and of Malaria Eradication*, Geneva, World Health Organization, 1963.

Fig. 4.5: Based, with small modifications, on a figure in A. P. Hall, The treatment of severe falciparum malaria, *Trans R Soc Trop Med Hyg* 71:367-379, 1977.

Fig. 4.6, 4.7: Based, with modifications, on figures by Dr. Marcos Boulos.

Fig 4.9: Based on a figure in K. M. Loban and E. S. Polozok, *Malaria*, Moscow, Mir Publishers, 1985.

Fig. 5.1, 5.2, 5.3, 5.5, 5.12, 5.23: Reproduced from the *Manual for the Microscopic Diagnosis of Malaria*, 4th ed., Washington, D.C., Pan American Health Organization, 1973.

Fig. 5.4, 5.6, 5.7, 5.8, 5.9, 5.10, 5.11, 5.13, 5.14, 5.15, 5.16, 5.17, 5.18, 5.19, 5.20, 5.21, 5.22, 5.24, 5.25, 5.26, 5.27: Drawn by Dr. F. J. López-Antuñano.

Fig. 5.5: Sketches B) and C) done by Dr. F. J. López-Antuñano from cerebral sections provided by Dr. A. Céspedes, pathologist at San Juan de Dios Hospital, San José, Costa Rica.

Fig. 6.1: Drawn by Dr. Janine Ramsey.

Fig. 7.1: Provided by Dr. Fidel Zavala.

Fig. 9.1, 9.2, 9.3, 9.4, 9.5: Reproduced from the *Manual for the Microscopic Diagnosis of Malaria*, 4th ed., Washington, D.C., Pan American Health Organization, 1973.

Fig. 9.6: Originally published in F. J. López-Antuñano, Microscopia en la malaria humana, *Boletín CNEP* No. 1, Año III, Supplement, January-March 1959, Mexico.

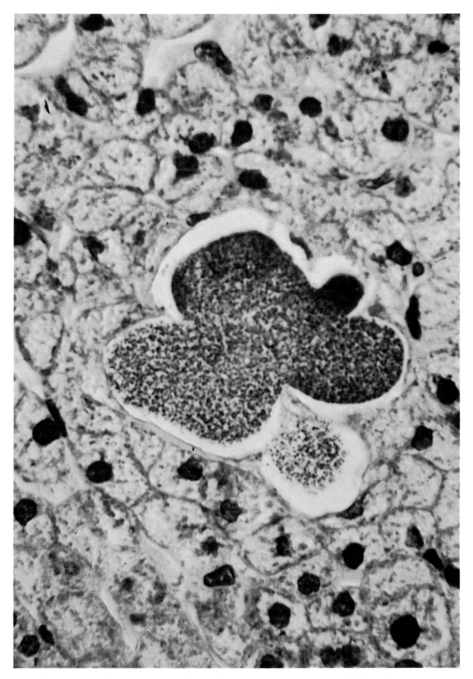

Figure 1.1. Histologic section of a liver biopsy from an individual with a seven-day-old *P. vivax* infection. The schizont is seen inside a liver cell.

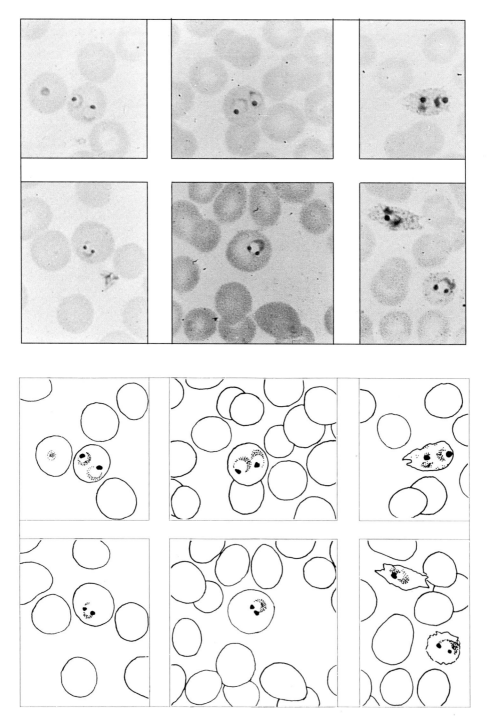

Figure 2.1. Morphology of ring forms of *Plasmodium falciparum, P. vivax,* and *P. ovale* in blood smears (from left to right).

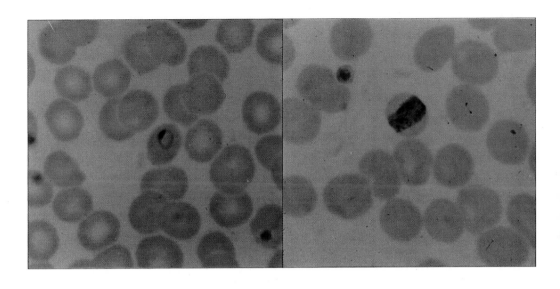

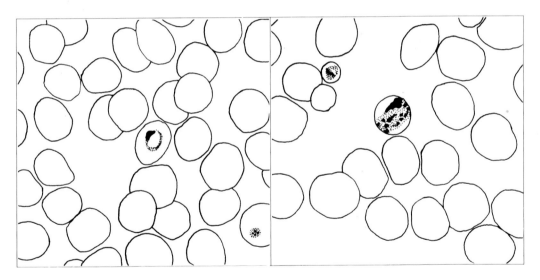

Figure 2.2. Morphology of ring and band forms of *Plasmodium malariae* in blood smears.

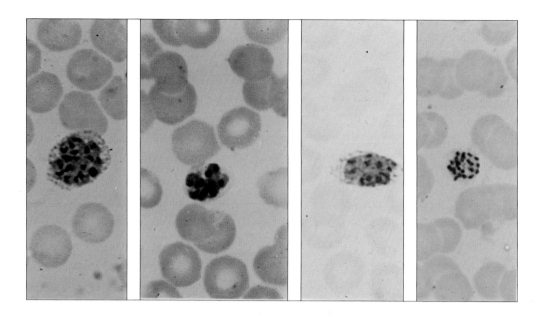

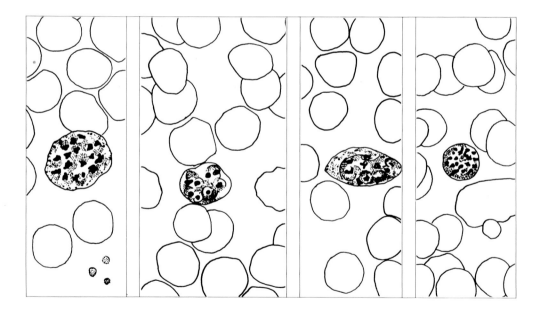

Figure 2.3. Morphology of the schizonts of *Plasmodium vivax, P. malariae, P. ovale,* and *P. falciparum* in blood smears (from left to right).

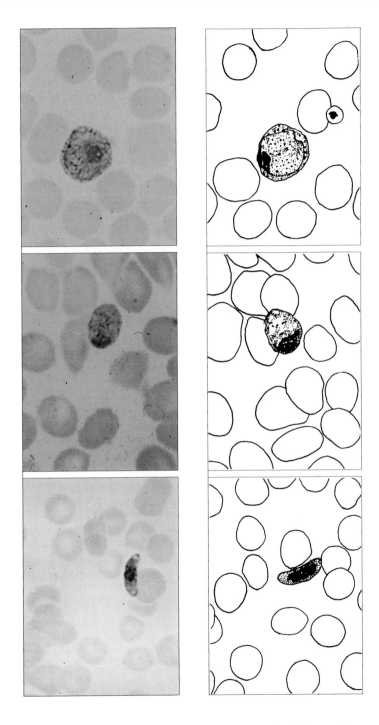

Figure 2.4. Morphology of the gametocytes of *Plasmodium vivax, P. malariae,* and *P. falciparum* in blood smears (from top to bottom).

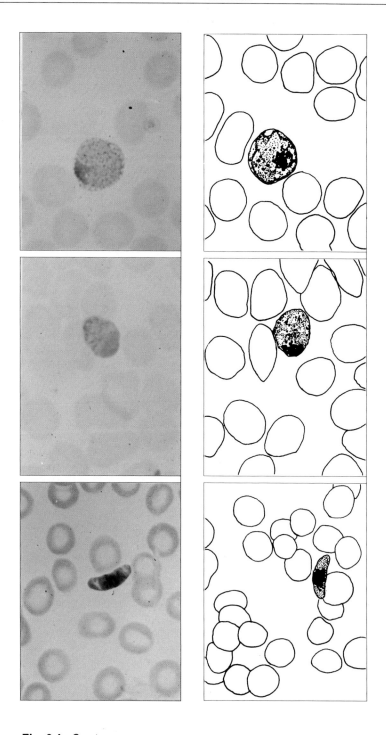

Fig. 2.4. *Cont.*

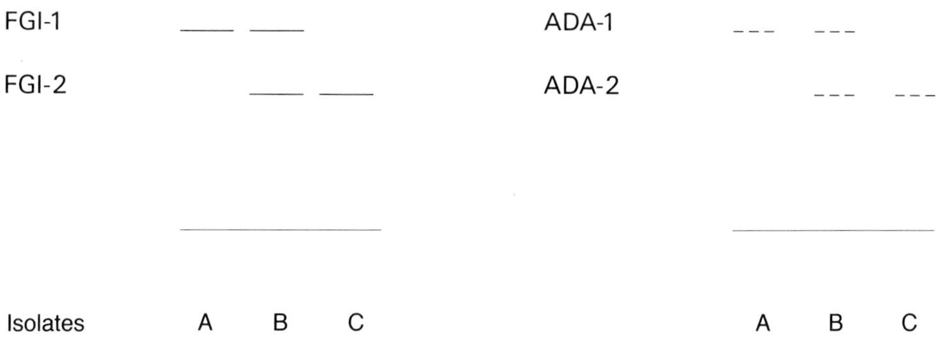

FGI-1   ____ ____   ADA-1   _ _ _   _ _ _

FGI-2   ____ ____   ADA-2   _ _ _   _ _ _

                    _____   _____

Isolates   A   B   C   A   B   C

        Isolate A = Homogeneous population of parasites of genotype GPI-1/ADA-1
        Isolate C = Homogeneous population of parasites of genotype GPI-2/ADA-2
        Isolate B = Heterogeneous population of parasites of:
                    a) mixture of genotypes GPI-1/ADA-1 and GPI-2/ADA-2
             or   b) mixture of genotypes GPI-1/ADA-2 and GPI-2/ADA-1
             or   c) mixture of genotypes GPI-1/ADA-1 and GPI-1/ADA-2 and GPI-2/ADA-1
             or   d) previous population (c) plus genotype GPI-2/ADA-2

Figure 2.5. Enzyme typing of *P. falciparum* from three isolates. Parasites from patients A, B, and C were maintained in culture until a 3% parasitemia with predominance of schizonts was obtained. These parasites were concentrated and prepared for glucose phosphate isomerase (GPI) and adenosine deaminase (ADA) typing using cellulose acetate electrophoresis. Isolate A comprises a population of parasites of type GPI-1, ADA-1. Isolate C also comprises a homogeneous population of parasites, different from isolate A, of type GPI-2, ADA-2. Isolate B, however, is a mixture of parasites, since two different types for each enzyme were observed, corresponding to four different possibilities of simultaneous growth of different parasites. Only cloning would properly identify each parasite population.

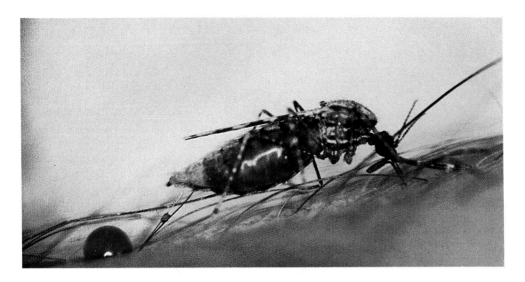

Figure 3.1. *Anopheles stephensi*, a prinicpal malaria vector in Asia, feeding on a human host. (Note the large fluid droplet excreted while ingesting and concentrating the blood meal.)

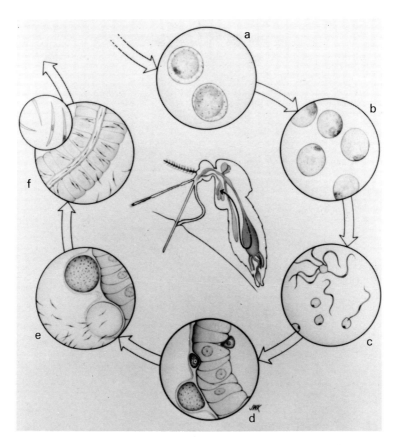

Figure 3.2. The development cycle of a malaria parasite (*Plasmodium vivax*) in the mosquito gut. (a) Macro- and microgametocytes ingested with the blood meal by the mosquito. (b) Gametocytes freed from erythrocytes in the mosquito midgut. (c) Exflagellation, the release of spermlike microgametes in the mosquito midgut. (d) Ookinetes penetrating the wall of the mosquito midgut and initiation of oocyst development under the basal membrane of the gut. (e) Oocyst on the mosquito gut and release of sporozoites into the hemocoel. (f) Sporozoites penetrating the salivary gland.

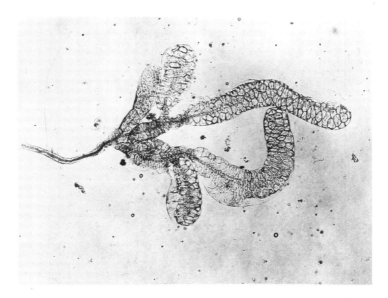

Figure 3.3. Salivary glands of a mosquito. Each of the paired glands consists of three lobes.

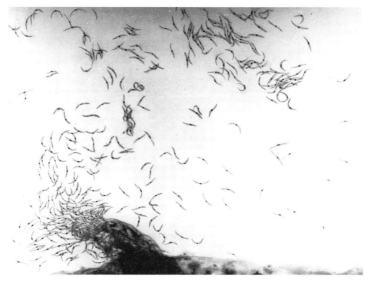

Figure 3.4. Sporozoites released from a heavily infected salivary gland of a mosquito.

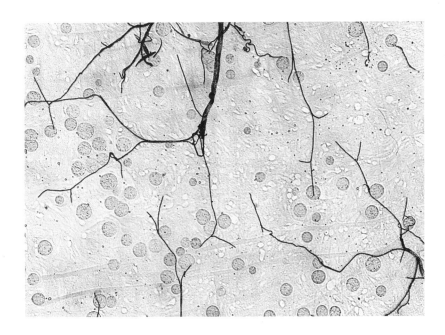

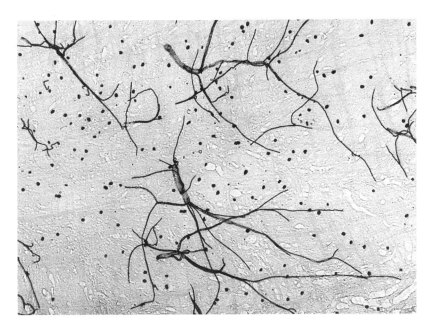

Figure 3.5. Top: Oocysts growing on the gut of *Anopheles gambiae* mosquito, six days after an infectious blood meal. Bottom: Encapsulated oocysts on the gut of a genetically selected refractory *Anopheles gambiae* mosquito. No sporozoites will develop from these oocysts.

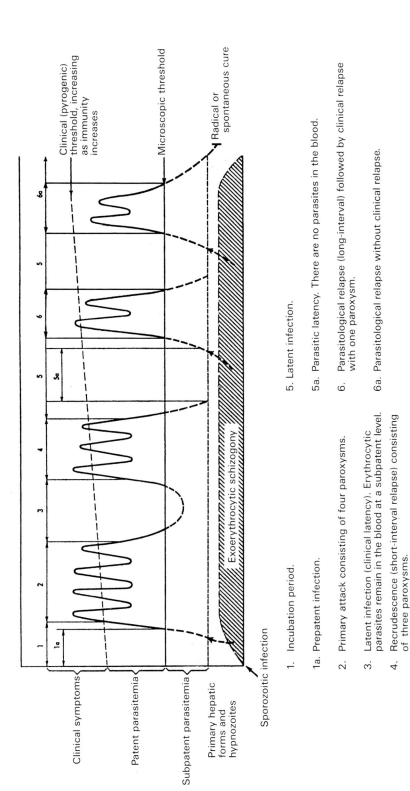

Figure 4.1. Phases of a malarial infection, indicating recrudescences and relapses.

1. Incubation period.

1a. Prepatent infection.

2. Primary attack consisting of four paroxysms.

3. Latent infection (clinical latency). Erythrocytic parasites remain in the blood at a subpatent level.

4. Recrudescence (short-interval relapse) consisting of three paroxysms.

5. Latent infection.

5a. Parasitic latency. There are no parasites in the blood.

6. Parasitological relapse (long-interval) followed by clinical relapse with one paroxysm.

6a. Parasitological relapse without clinical relapse.

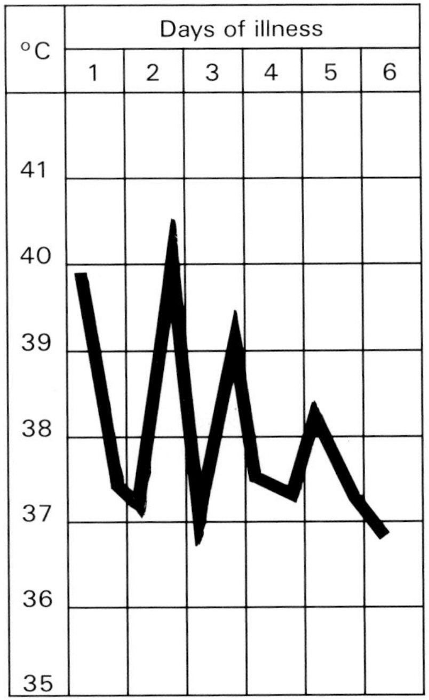

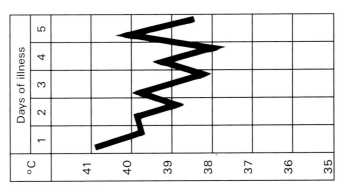

Figure 4.4. Continuous fever caused by *P. falciparum*.

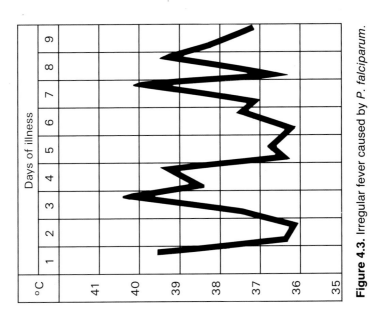

Figure 4.3. Irregular fever caused by *P. falciparum*.

Figure 4.2. Daily intermittent fever caused by *P. falciparum*.

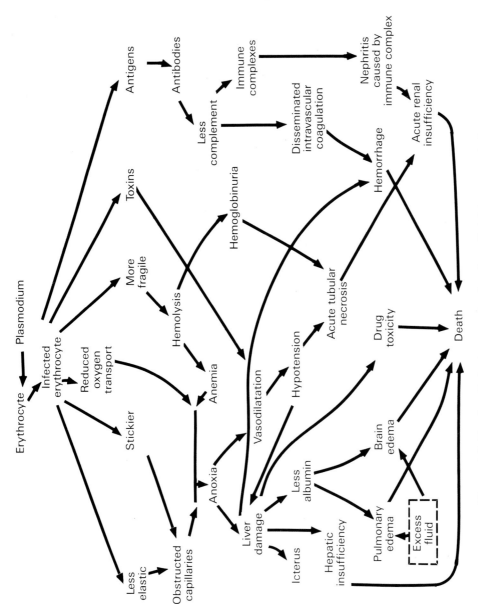

Figure 4.5. Physiopathologic cascade of serious *P. falciparum* malaria.

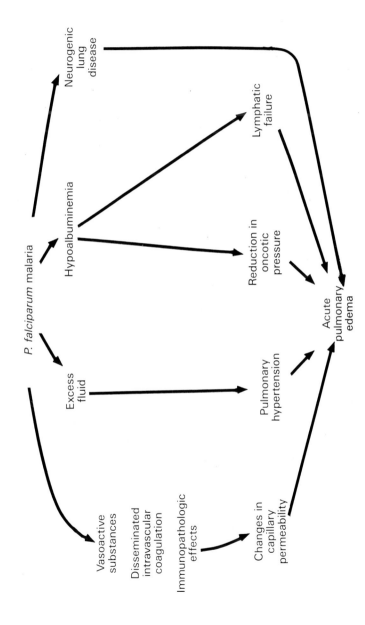

Figure 4.6. Physiopathology of acute pulmonary edema in *P. falciparum* malaria.

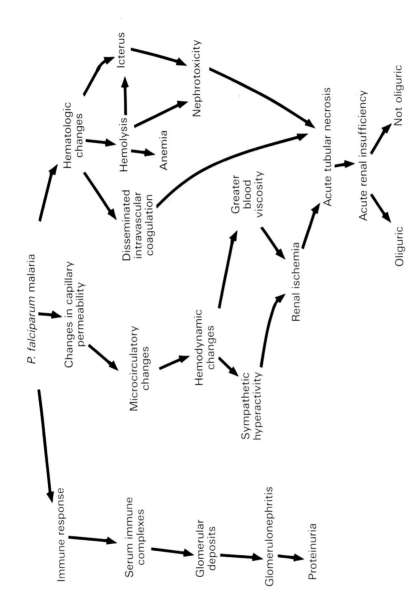

Figure 4.7. Physiopathology of renal insufficiency in *P. falciparum* malaria.

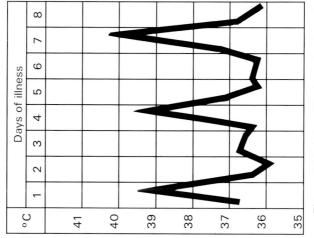

Figure 4.10. Intermittent quartan fever in *P. malariae* malaria.

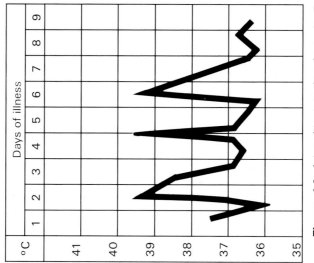

Figure 4.9. Intermittent tertian fever in *P. ovale* malaria.

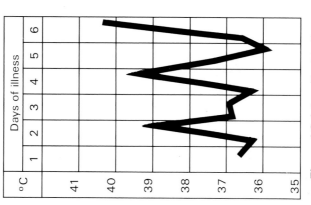

Figure 4.8. Intermittent tertian fever in *P. vivax* malaria.

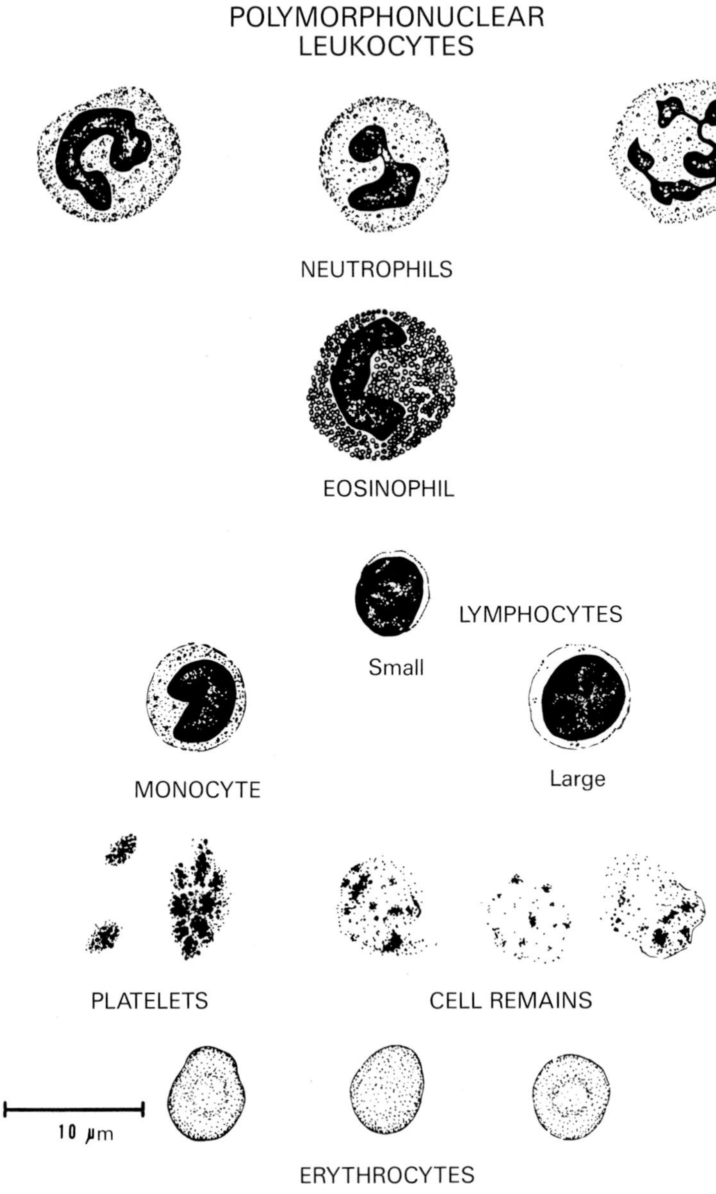

POLYMORPHONUCLEAR
LEUKOCYTES

NEUTROPHILS

EOSINOPHIL

LYMPHOCYTES

Small

MONOCYTE

Large

PLATELETS   CELL REMAINS

10 µm

ERYTHROCYTES

Figure 5.1. Characteristics and sizes of some blood elements usually seen in the examination of a thick film.

Figure 5.2. Release of *P. falciparum* merozoites from a mature schizont and growth of the ring forms. These are the only asexual forms commonly encountered in the peripheral blood. The older asexual forms complete their growth in red blood cells that adhere to the capillaries of various organs, and are therefore not illustrated here. Occasionally, in very severe *P. falciparum* infections, fully developed schizonts may be seen in the peripheral blood. The *in vivo* growth course of *P. falciparum* gametocytes (indicated by the broken arrow) is unknown; although they originate from the erythrocytic merozoites, the mature sexual forms appear in the circulation only after two or three weeks of infection.

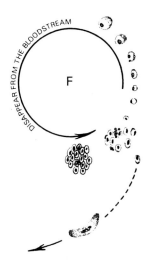

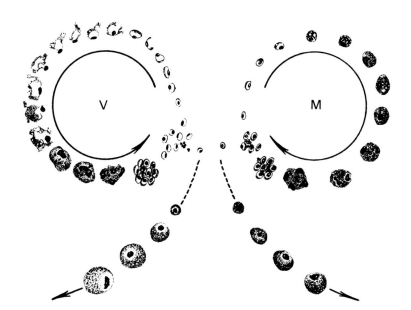

Figure 5.3. Erythrocytic cycle of *P. vivax* and *P. malariae*. After release of the merozoites from the mature schizont, the asexual stages continue their growth in the peripheral blood. The young ring forms of these two species as well as *P. falciparum* are practically indistinguishable. As they grow, however, *P. vivax* generally shows great pseudopodal activity within the red blood cell, while asexual forms of *P. malariae* give the impression of remaining stable and undisturbed and hence regular in shape. The gametocytes of these two species have development patterns completely different from those of the asexual forms.

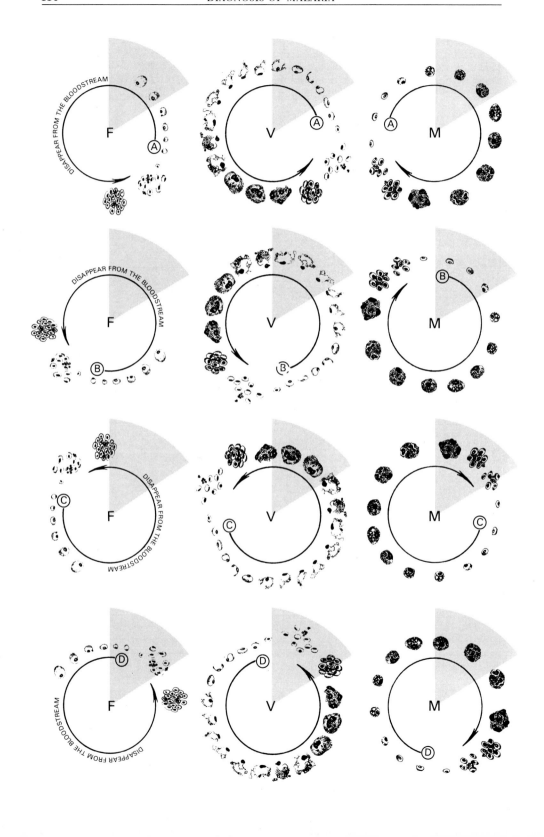

Figure 5.4. (Left) Broods. The cycles marked F (*P. falciparum*), V (*P. vivax*), and M (*P. malariae*) represent schematically the evolution of four broods (A, B, C, D) of those three species. The circular arrow indicates the direction the development cycle is proceeding in the sketch; the shaded angle shows what portion of the population of parasites of each brood or schizogony would be most numerous at a given moment.

For example, in a blood sample taken at the moment illustrated from a patient infected with *P. falciparum*, a few small ring forms corresponding to brood D would be observed, but there would also be some large rings from brood A; no parasites from broods B and C would be seen. However, even though few parasites would be found, the patient could still be gravely ill. In the case of *P. vivax* infection, practically the entire erythrocytic cycle will probably be seen in only one blood specimen if two or more broods are present: small rings from brood D mixed with large rings and small irregular forms from brood A, large irregular forms from B, and large mononuclear parasites and schizonts from brood C. In *P. malariae* infections, the ring forms of brood B can be observed together with the compact, pigmented, regular forms from brood A, schizonts from brood C, and large mononuclear parasites and schizonts from D.

The brood phenomenon is very important not only in understanding parasite variation for purposes of specific diagnosis but, more importantly, for evaluating a patient's condition.

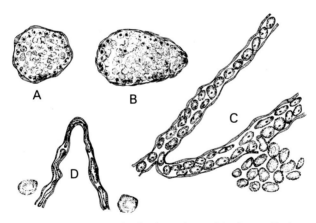

Figure 5.5. Transverse and longitudinal sections of brain capillaries containing erythrocytes parasitized by *P. falciparum*.

A) Transverse section of a cerebral capillary.

B) Transverse section of a venule in the brain of a fatal case. The red blood cells containing mature parasites and malarial pigment are stuck to the vessel endothelium.

C) Longitudinal section of a capillary. One of its branches has a damaged site through which uninfected red blood cells or those containing very young parasites (rings) exit. The black dots represent the parasites inside erythrocytes adhering to the capillary.

D) Unparasitized red blood cells, which are very elastic, easily traverse the capillary lumen by adapting their shape to the shape of the blood vessel wall.

Figure 5.6. Scarce small rings of *P. falciparum*.

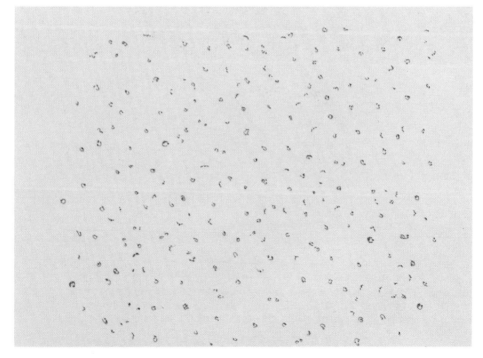

Figure 5.7. Very abundant small rings of *P. falciparum*.

Figure 5.8. Scarce medium-sized rings of *P. falciparum*.

Figure 5.9. Abundant medium-sized rings of *P. falciparum*.

Figure 5.10. Scarce large rings of *P. falciparum*.

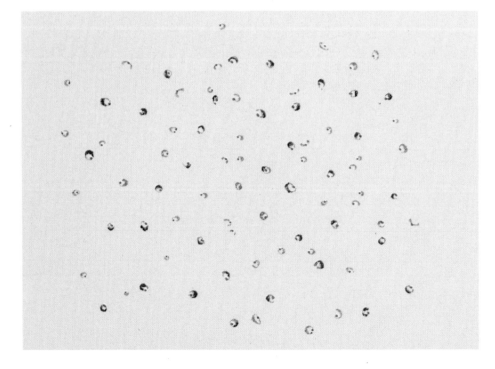

Figure 5.11. Abundant large rings of *P. falciparum*.

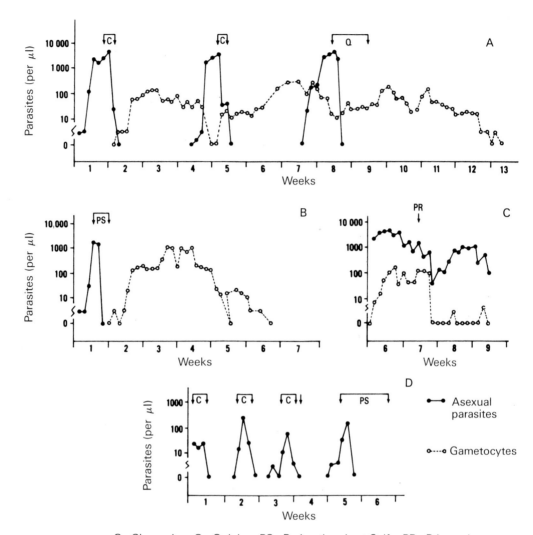

C=Cloroquine; Q=Quinine; PS=Pyrimethamine+Sulfa; PR=Primaquine

Figure 5.12. Typical behavior patterns of *P. falciparum* gametocytes.

A) Appearance of gametocytes during the second week of patent asexual parasitemia; the asexual parasitemia is reduced after two treatments with chloroquine but is only eliminated after a third treatment with quinine. The gametocytes are present from the second week of patent infection and persist during weeks 8 through 13 despite the fact that the patient's clinical symptoms have been cured.

B) Appearance of gametocytes as in A), and their spontaneous depletion five weeks after treatment with pyrimethamine and sulfadoxine.

C) Simultaneous presence of asexual forms and gametocytes during the sixth and seventh weeks of infection. Elimination of circulating gametocytes after treatment with primaquine.

D) Prevention of gametocytocemia by means of administration of schizonticides as soon as the asexual forms become patent.

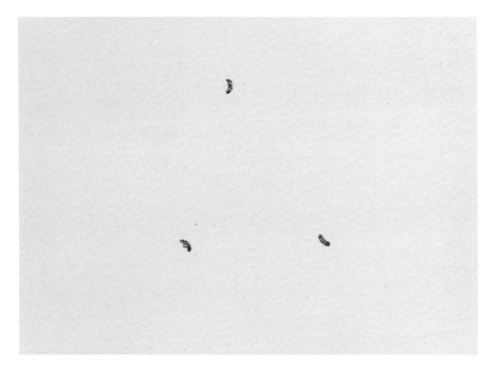

Figure 5.13. Scarce gametocytes of *P. falciparum*.

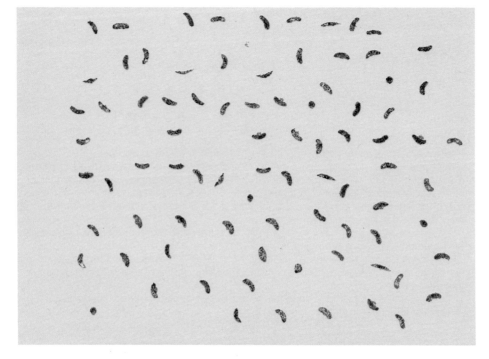

Figure 5.14. Abundant gametocytes of *P. falciparum*.

Figure 5.15. Scarce forms of *P. vivax*; most are ring forms.

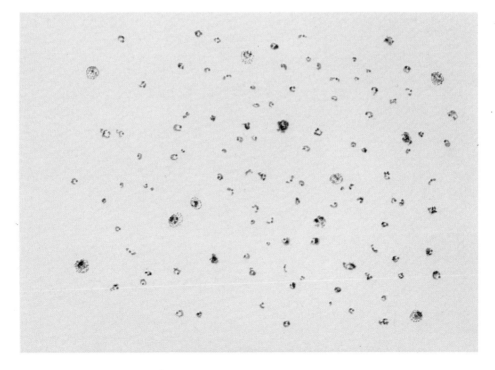

Figure 5.16. Abundant forms of *P. vivax*; most are ring forms.

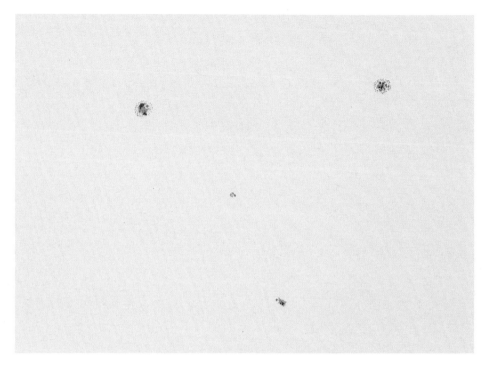

Figure 5.17. Scarce forms of *P. vivax*; most are irregular forms.

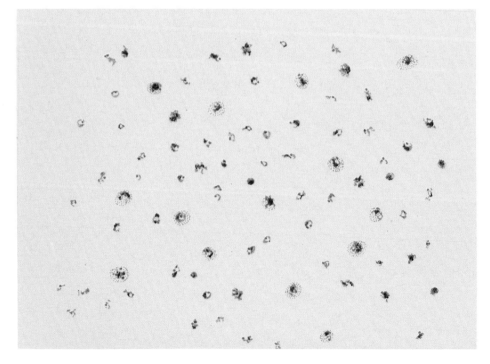

Figure 5.18. Abundant forms of *P. vivax*; most are irregular forms.

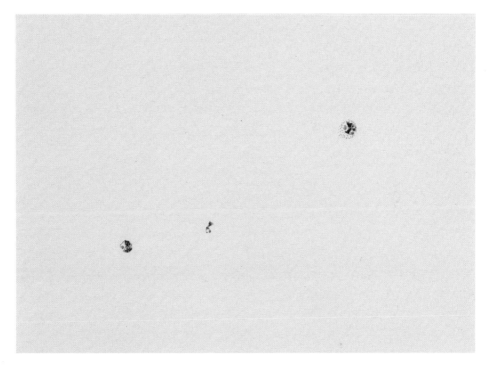

Figure 5.19. Scarce forms of *P. vivax*; it is difficult to determine which forms predominate.

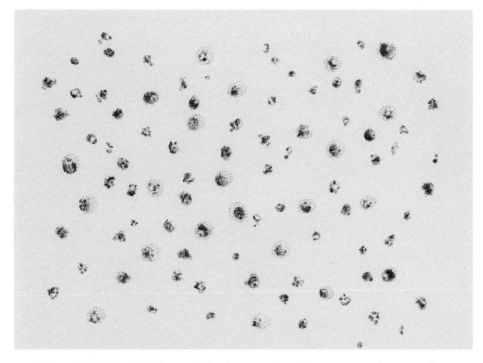

Figure 5.20. Abundant forms of *P. vivax*; most are large mononuclear parasites.

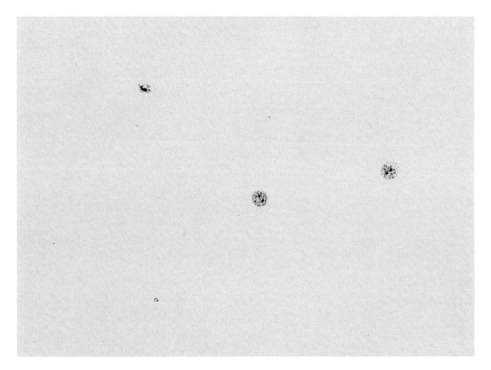

Figure 5.21. Scarce forms of *P. vivax*; most are schizonts.

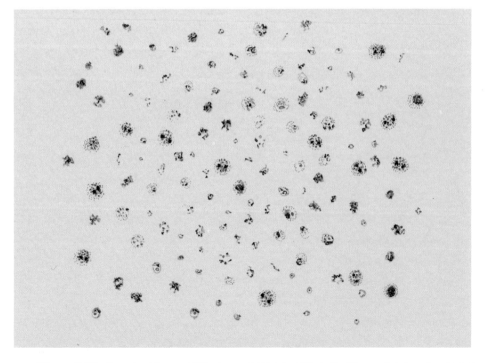

Figure 5.22. Abundant forms of *P. vivax*; most are schizonts. The numerous ring forms signal the beginning of the next schizogony.

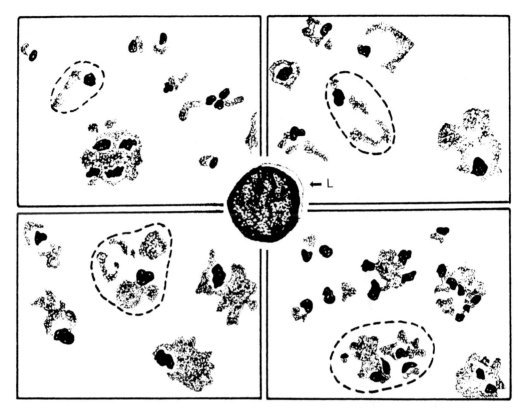

Figure 5.23. Use of a nearby small lymphocyte (L) to gauge the surface area covered by an entire parasite.

Figure 5.24. Scarce forms of *P. malariae*; it is difficult to determine which forms predominate.

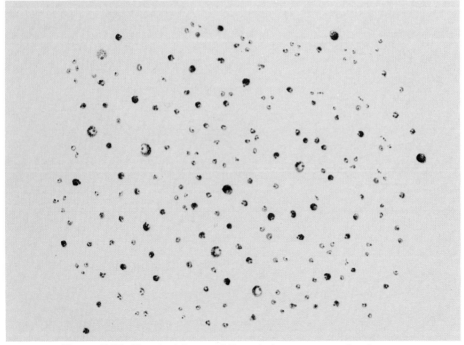

Figure 5.25. Abundant forms of *P. malariae*; most are ring forms.

Figure 5.26. Scarce forms of *P. malariae*; it is difficult to determine which forms predominate.

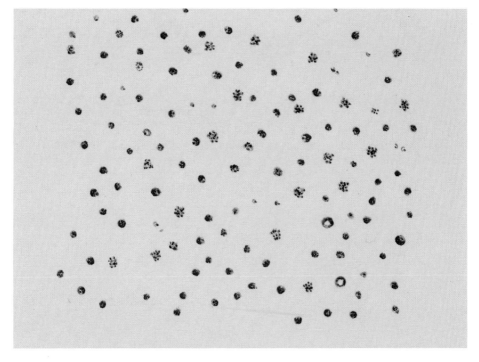

Figure 5.27. Abundant forms of *P. malariae*; most are compact parasites with a high concentration of pigment. This example shows many schizonts with few merozoites.

Dissection of Midgut

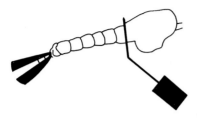

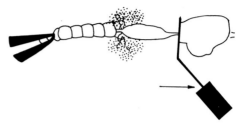

1. Pin with forceps at the seventh segment. Place needle at thorax-abdomen joint.

2. Pull to right with needle pressed slightly downward.

Dissection of Salivary Glands

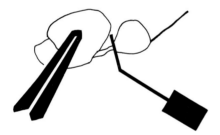

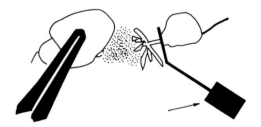

1. Exert downward pressure with forceps.

2. Pull needle to right with downward pressure, severing the gland connection in the same movement.

Figure 6.1. Dissection of midgut and salivary glands of mosquitoes in order to look for malaria parasites.

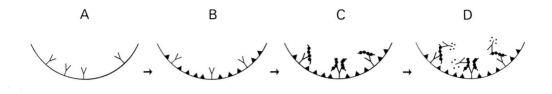

Y	Monoclonal antibody
▲	Nonspecific protein
⋏	Sporozoite antigen
⋏	Labeled monoclonal antibody

Figure 7.1. Schematic representation of the different steps of the two-site immunoassay. A) The monoclonal antibody adheres to the plastic. B) To saturate the binding sites on the surface of the plastic, another protein is added (casein or albumin). C) The antibody, immobilized on the plate, binds antigen. D) The bound antigen still has free antigenic determinants that bind labeled antibodies.

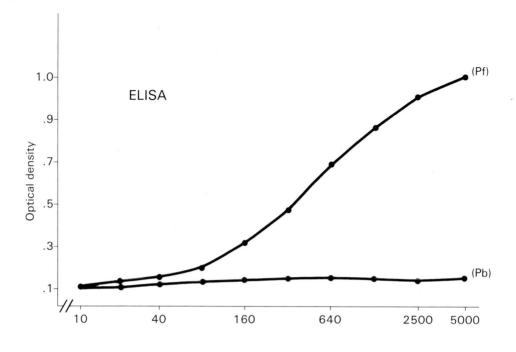

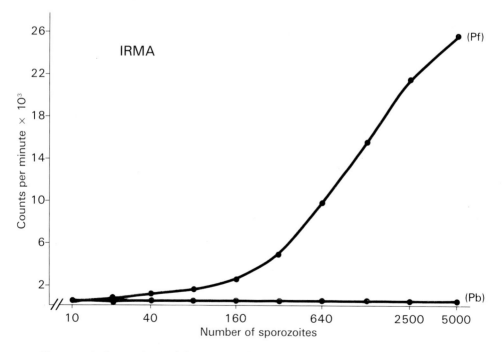

Figure 7.2. Comparison of the results obtained by IRMA and ELISA for detection of *P. falciparum* sporozoites. The same *P. falciparum* sporozoite extract (Pf) containing a known number of parasites was used to perform both assays simultaneously. As a negative control an extract of *P. berghei* sporozoites (Pb) was used.

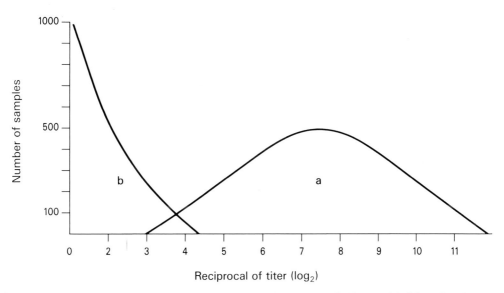

Figure 8.1. Distribution frequency curves of titers in individuals with (a) and without (b) malarial antibodies, as found using the indirect hemagglutination test.

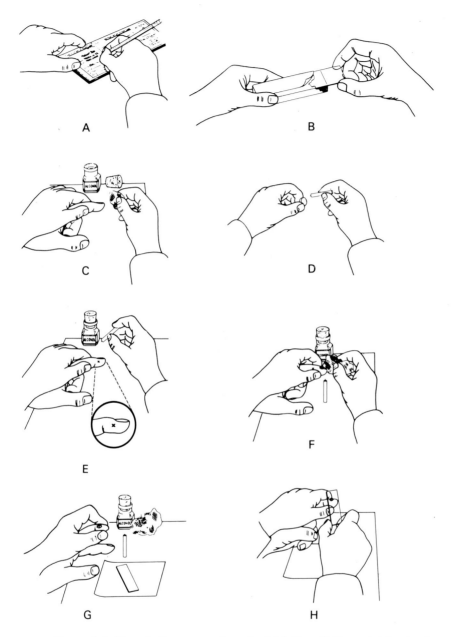

Figure 9.1. Steps in the preparation of a thick film. A) Record data about patient. B) Take out a slide. C) Cleanse the site to be punctured. D) Use disposable lancet or needle. E) Prick the patient's finger. F) Wipe off the first drop of blood. G) Press the finger to obtain another drop. H) Deposit the blood on the slide. I) With a second slide, spread the blood into a square or oval of

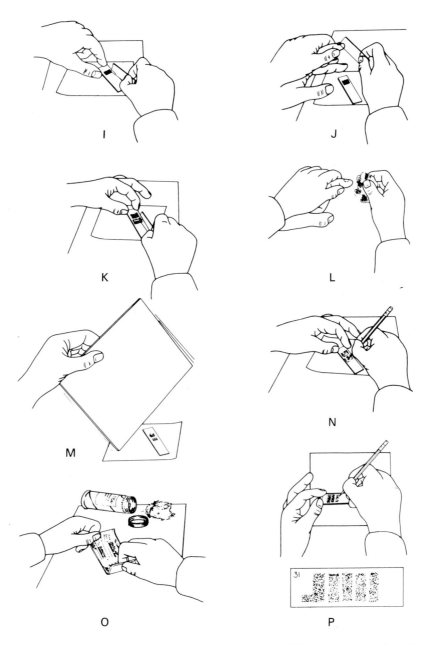

appropriate size. J), K) Using the same spreader slide, put another drop of blood on the first slide. L) Clean the finger with alcohol. M) Place the slide containing the blood samples on a flat surface and allow it to dry. N) Write identification on the slide. O) Wrap the sample. P) Illustration of the pattern for arranging multiple samples.

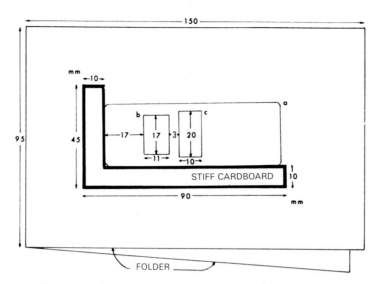

Figure 9.2. Guide for positioning a thick film (b) and an identification label (c) on a slide (a).

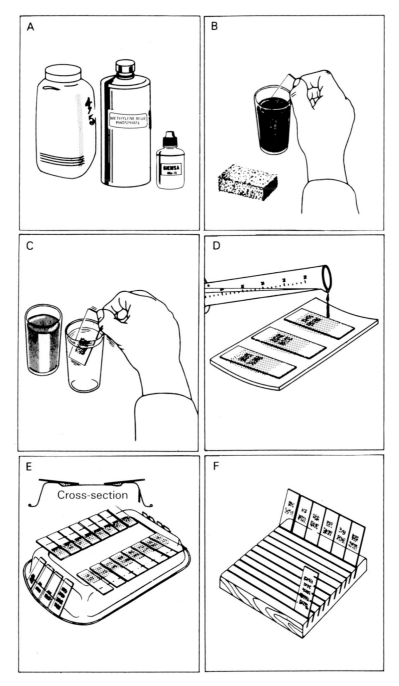

Figure 9.3. Main steps of Walker's method for staining thick blood films. A) Illustration of set of containers for mixing solutions. B) Dip slide in methylene blue phosphate solution. C) Rinse the slide in buffer solution. D) Allow the stain to flow under slides inverted on a concave plate. E) For a larger number of slides, do staining procedure on an enameled tray bottom. F) Set slides in a grooved rack to dry.

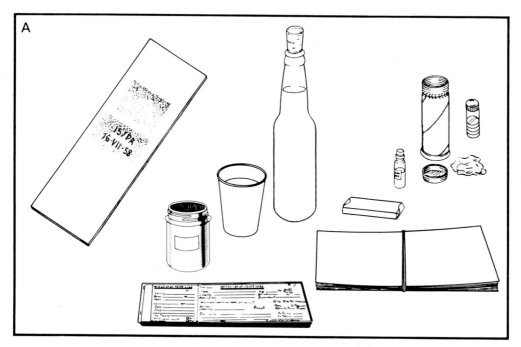

Figure 9.4. Detailed description of the first step of Walker's method for staining thick blood films.

A) All the necessary materials are gathered: the unstained thick film sample; wide-mouthed bottle filled with methylene blue phosphate solution; small glass and thoroughly washed bottle containing 300 ml distilled water; cardboard box for shipping slides; buffer salts; antimalarial drugs; pad of forms for notification of febrile cases; and packet of paper for wrapping the slides.

B) Empty the buffer salts into the distilled water.

C) Once the salts have dissolved, fill the glass two-thirds full with the solution.

D) Holding the slide by the end opposite the sample, submerse it for one second in the methylene blue solution.

E) Let the excess methylene blue drain off the slide.

F) Immediately dip the slide in the glass containing the buffer solution and gently stir until the borders of the sample begin to lose their red color. When the buffer solution begins to turn deep blue, it should be replaced with fresh solution from the bottle. The methylene blue solution can be reused repeatedly. Buffered methylene blue should be kept in a tightly sealed bottle and can be used for up to six months.

G) Lean the slide against a suitable support where it can drain and dry. After this step, the slide should appear almost transparent.

H) In cases where it is not possible to proceed immediately to the second step of Walker's method, wrap the dry slide in paper and, with the notification report, leave for later processing or send to a laboratory for staining and microscopic observation.

I) If the patient shows the characteristic symptoms, administer antimalarial drugs.

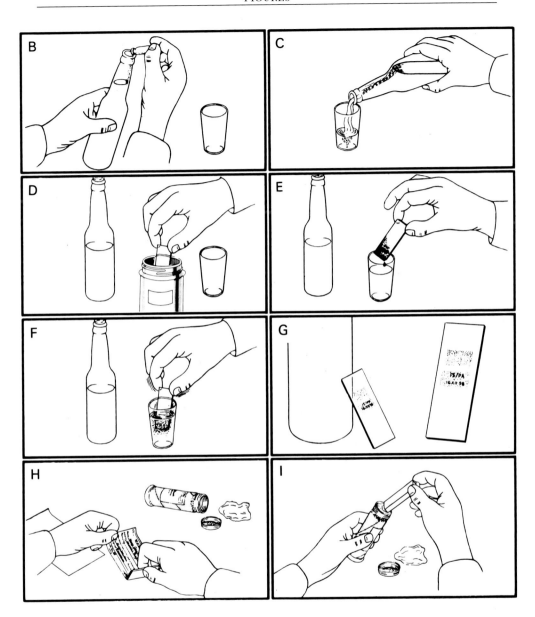

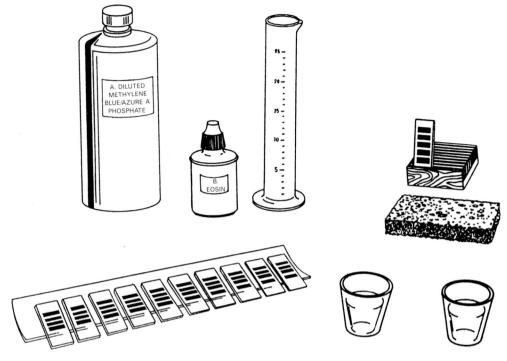

Figure 9.5. Romanowsky's method (modified) for staining a thick blood film.

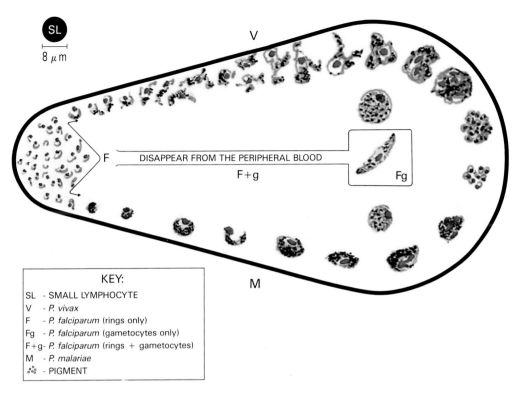

KEY:
SL - SMALL LYMPHOCYTE
V   - *P. vivax*
F   - *P. falciparum* (rings only)
Fg - *P. falciparum* (gametocytes only)
F+g- *P. falciparum* (rings + gametocytes)
M   - *P. malariae*
•°• - PIGMENT

Figure 9.6. The appearance in a thick film of different species of human plasmodia in different stages of their erythrocytic cycle.